BAILLIÈR
SELF-ASSESSMENT

Revise General
Nursing
2

Other books by the same authors:

Revise General Nursing 1 covers the following topics:

- Care of the patient with problems of the heart and circulation
- Care of the patient with an endocrine disorder
- Care of the patient with problems of the alimentary and biliary tracts
- Care of the patient with a mental or physical handicap
- Care of the patient with problems of bones and joints

Revise General Nursing 3 covers the following topics:

- Care of the patient with respiratory problems
- Care of the highly dependent patient
- Care of the patient with problems of body image
- Care of the sick child
- Care of the patient with problems of the nervous system

Baillière's Nursing Study Aids *Crosswords for Revision*—30 crosswords to help students learn, covering the following topics:

Abdominal surgery; anaemia; ante-natal care; anorexia nervosa; asthma; cardiac failure; cerebrovascular accident; cholecystitis; chronic bronchitis; Crohn's disease; community care; diabetes mellitus; eczema; fractured femur; head injury; leukaemia; mastectomy; meningitis; myocardial infarction; nephrotic syndrome; non-accidental injury; paediatric gastroenteritis; peptic ulcer; psoriasis; pyloric stenosis; renal failure; rheumatoid arthritis; thyroidectomy; tonsillectomy; vaginal hysterectomy.

BAILLIÈRE'S
SELF-ASSESSMENT FOR NURSES

Revise General Nursing 2

Christina Cheetham
SRN, RSCN, RCNT, Cert. Ed., RNT
Senior Tutor
Charles West School of Nursing
Great Ormond St, London

Joan Ramsay
SRN, DN(Lond.), Cert. Ed., RNT
Senior Tutor
Charles West School of Nursing
Great Ormond St, London

Baillière Tindall
London   Philadelphia   Toronto
Sydney   Tokyo   Hong Kong

Baillière Tindall 33 The Avenue
W. B. Saunders Eastbourne, East Sussex BN21 3UN, England

West Washington Square
Philadelphia, PA 19105, USA

1 Goldthorne Avenue
Toronto, Ontario M8Z 5T9, Canada

ABP Australia Ltd, 44–50 Waterloo Road
North Ryde, NSW 2113, Australia

Ichibancho Central Building, 22–1 Ichibancho
Chiyoda-ku, Tokyo 102, Japan

10/fl, Inter-Continental Plaza, 94 Granville Road
Tsim Sha Tsui East, Kowloon, Hong Kong

First published 1987

Typeset by Photo·graphics
Printed and bound in Great Britain by Biddles Ltd,
Guildford, Surrey

British Library Cataloguing in Publication Data
Cheetham, Christina
  Revise general nursing 2.—
  (Baillière's self-assessment for nurses)
  1. Nursing—Problems, exercises, etc.
  I. Title II. Ramsay, Joan III. Series
  610.73′076   RT55

  ISBN 0–7020–1193–2

Contents

Preface

The aim of this series of books is to provide the learner with an active means of independently evaluating his/her knowledge and understanding of patient care.

The books are intended for RGN students as a way of consolidating their previous knowledge. They could be used at the end of each unit of learning or as an aid to revision at the end of training.

It is probable that with the recent development of the state final examination, individual hospitals will have differing methods of assessment. However, whatever form of assessment is used, these books should provide a useful means for the learner to evaluate his/her own knowledge and understanding.

The three books are all sub-divided into five chapters, each concerned with a particular patient problem. The wide range of experience encountered by the learner during her training is covered within these chapters. Each chapter consists of a number of short case-histories and related questions.

The questions are concerned with the assessment, planning, implementation and evaluation of individual patients' care. The concepts of holistic nursing and research are seen as important aspects throughout. Suggested answers to questions are given after each case history.

Application of knowledge and problem-solving is seen as more important than recall of facts. This form of revision ensures that the learner understands the rationale for nursing care, and is able to be adaptable in different situations.

Acknowledgement must be made to the support and invaluable assistance given by Ms Richenda Milton-Thompson of Baillière Tindall.

Thanks also go to Mrs Susanne Walker and Mrs Maggie Wisby for typing the manuscript.

C. Cheetham

J. Ramsay

Introduction:
How to Use this Book

- This book has been designed to help you learn by yourself. You will find that it is divided into five chapters, each relating to a particular patient problem. Some you will have come across already; some you may meet later in your career. You might prefer to look at the problems you are familiar with first, as the sections do not interrelate, and can be taken in any order.
- The book is primarily intended as a consolidation of your previous theoretical and practical experiences. Therefore, you may wish to do some preparatory reading or revision before you tackle any of the case-histories. You may also use them as a pre-test of your knowledge. You may know more than you think!
- Questions are worded differently. To help you decide the most appropriate way to answer each you may like to spend some time familiarizing yourself with the commonly used words as shown below:

  Define: to state precisely your meaning of
  Describe: to give an account or representation of, in your own words
  Discuss: to investigate, examine by argument (i.e. by logical discussion), to sift or debate ideas and to reach your conclusion
  Explain: to make plain, interpret or account for; to give the reasons for your actions
  Identify: to determine the individual characteristics of
  List: to give an item-by-item record
  Outline: to provide a draft account, giving the main reasons or general principles of a subject
  State: to present in a brief, concise format
- The style of your answers is entirely up to you. You do not have to write a timed essay; notes will do. However, we do suggest some kind of written response as educational research shows that this significantly improves memory. Any help in remembering must be worth using!

- Do not worry if your answers are slightly different to those given. Our answers are not intended to be the only correct ones, but do contain the essential points. Also, we realize that each hospital has its own local practices. You may have to adapt our answer to meet your own hospital procedure.
- You will find that some topics are very specialized. If you have not had experience in these specialities you may prefer to use such case-histories to extend your knowledge rather than as a basis for revision.
- You will also find that some questions in some case-histories relate to ward management and teaching junior colleagues. You may wish to omit these questions until you have had experience in these areas.
- We hope that you find this way of studying useful, and, most importantly, enjoyable! If so, you may be interested in the companion volumes to this book.

1 Care of the Elderly Patient

1.1   Miss Grange—an elderly patient with anaemia

Miss Edith Grange, aged 80 years, has been admitted for investigations of anaemia. She has been referred by her general practitioner who discovered that she had a haemoglobin concentration of 5 g/l.

Miss Grange lives in a warden-controlled flat. She is a very independent lady who is very reluctant to come into hospital. She originally visited her doctor thinking that she needed a tonic to help her persistent tiredness, never imagining that he would suggest admission to hospital.

1   State the possible reasons for Miss Grange's reluctance to be admitted. How might these reasons be overcome?

2   Giving reasons, what specific information is needed from Miss Grange on admission in order to plan her care?

3   With reference to normal and altered physiology explain anaemia and its three main causes.

4   Describe the role of the nurse when caring for Miss Grange before, during and after:
   (a) a bone marrow puncture
   (b) a Schilling test

Miss Grange is diagnosed as having pernicious anaemia. Her bone marrow puncture results show immature, hypochromic, macrocytic red cells. Cyanocobalamin is prescribed, and in view of her low haemoglobin level she is also to have a blood transfusion.

5   With reference to normal physiology explain Miss Grange's blood results and diagnosis to a junior nurse.

6   What will be Miss Grange's actual and potential problems during her blood transfusion and what actions should be taken to overcome these problems?

7   What advice should Miss Grange receive on discharge?

1.1   Answers

1

Possible reasons for reluctance	Methods to overcome these problems
Loss of independence	• Show Miss Grange around the ward. • Involve her in planning her care. • Allow her to be as independent as possible.
Loss of self-esteem	• Ask Miss Grange what she wishes to be called. • Allow her to get up and dressed.
Fear of illness and hospitals	• Explain all investigations and results as available. • Allow time for her to express any fears.
Loneliness/a strange environment	• Introduce other patients and staff. • Explain ward routine.

2

Information	Planning care
Breathing • Is Miss Grange breathless? • Is her dyspnoea obvious or does it only occur on exertion?	Miss Grange's mobility and ability to be independent may be affected by this. Four-hourly respirations may be indicated to assess any improvement or deterioration.
Eating and Drinking • What kind of diet does Miss Grange eat at home? (Is dietary deficiency of iron likely?)	Record her likes and dislikes
• Has she had any indigestion, loss of appetite or vomiting?	Special care may be needed in planning her diet if these features of anaemia are present.
• Does she have any soreness of her mouth or tongue?	

- Does she have any dental problems?

Loose or bad teeth may interfere with a proper dietary intake.

Excretion
- What is Miss Grange's normal bowel habit?
- What colour are her stools? (Is melaena a feature?)

The degree of constipation must be assessed (especially if iron is prescribed).

Sleep and rest
- How much sleep and rest does Miss Grange like to have?

Care can be planned not only to help Miss Grange with activities of daily living but also to allow for rest periods.

Vital signs
- Pulse—rate and rhythm?
- Has she had any palpitations?
- Skin colour?

Atrial fibrillation may be a complicating feature which will need monitoring.
A yellowish tinge to the skin may indicate pernicious anaemia.

- Has she noticed any ankle swelling?

Heart failure may develop from anaemia. Any oedema will need regular evaluation.

Special senses
- Does her hearing and vision appear normal? Does she wear glasses or a hearing aid?

Care can be planned to take into account any sensory deficit.

- Has she had any loss of balance, numbness or tingling of the hands or feet?

Subacute degeneration of the spinal cord can complicate vitamin B_{12} deficiency.

Such features would require the care plan to include the maintenance of safety.

Mobility
- Is Miss Grange active for her age or does she need help with some activities?

Help can be planned where necessary.

- Does she manage alone in her flat or does she have community services?

The care plan must take account of home circumstances so that discharge is realistic.

3   Red cells or erythrocytes perform the important function of carrying oxygen from the lungs to the tissues.

The number of red cells varies with age, sex and altitude. Normally, women average about 4 500 000 red blood cells per cubic millimetre of blood.

Oxygen is carried in the red cells by combining with haemoglobin—a protein found in the red cells. The average normal amount of haemoglobin is 14.5–15 g/100 ml blood.

Anaemia is a deficiency in either the quality or the quantity of red blood cells, resulting in below normal levels of circulating oxygen. The three main causes of anaemia are:
- Loss of red blood cells, i.e. haemorrhage
- Increased haemolysis
- Decreased production of erythrocytes

4 (a) **Bone marrow puncture**
- **Preparation** Explain to Miss Grange that a specimen of bone marrow is needed as this is where the red cells are produced. The bone marrow of her sternum (chest bone) will be used. A long needle will be inserted to withdraw the sample of tissue. Miss Grange may feel discomfort when the specimen is taken, as well as apprehension and a feeling of pressure when the needle is inserted. However, the procedure only takes about as long as an injection.
- **During the procedure** Provide a clean, dry dressing trolley and a dressing pack. Help Miss Grange into a comfortable position on her back and possibly hold her hand when the needle is inserted.
- **After the procedure** Ensure Miss Grange does not feel faint before adjusting her clothing and helping her up.

(b) **Schilling test**
- **Preparation** Explain to Miss Grange that she is to have an injection of vitamin B$_{12}$ followed by a drink containing vitamin B$_{12}$. Her urine is then collected for 24 hours. If her anaemia is caused by an inability to absorb vitamin B$_{12}$, very little of the vitamin will be excreted.
- **During the test** Ask Miss Grange to empty her bladder at the time you wish to commence the 24-hour collection. Discard this specimen. Collect all urine thereafter and the final specimen exactly 24 hours after your initial discard specimen. Ensure that all staff are aware of the need to save Miss Grange's urine. Ask her to use a labelled bedpan while the test is in progress.
- **After the procedure** Ensure that Miss Grange realizes that the test is complete.

5 Check the junior nurse's knowledge about the formation of

red cells. Explain to her how red cells mature: with the aid of a diagram such as that used in Fig. 1.

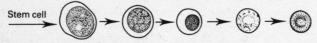

Proerythroblast Erythroblast Normoblast Reticulocyte Erythrocyte

Fig. 1   The development of red blood cells.

Miss Grange's red cells are large (macrocytic) and contain only small amounts of iron (hypochromic) and are thus identifiable as reticulocytes. This indicates a deficiency of one of the factors needed for red cell production. The junior nurse may be able to list these, thus:

- Iron
- Vitamin B_{12}
- Vitamin C
- Intrinsic factor
- Folic acid
- Healthy bone marrow

Vitamin B_{12} is necessary for the normal maturation of red cells. Miss Grange's red cells are immature so she must lack vitamin B_{12}. The body requires such a small amount of B_{12} that most people have adequate supply in their diet, e.g. in meat and diary products. Lack of vitamin B_{12} is caused by a lack of the intrinsic factor, found in the gastric juices, which is necessary for the absorption of vitamin B_{12}. This type of anaemia is called 'pernicious anaemia'.

6

Actual problems	Nursing actions
Reduced mobility—risk of pressure areas and deep vein thrombosis	• Help Miss Grange to move around and get up.
Inability to use one arm	• Wash Miss Grange daily. • Help with mouth cleaning and hair washing. • Cut up food.

Potential problems	Nursing actions
Incompatibility of transfusion	• Record pulse and BP hourly. • Report any tachycardia or hypotension. • Report any complaints of loin pain or anuria.

	• Check each unit of blood as hospital policy. Save all empty blood bags.
Pulmonary oedema—due to overloading circulation	• Check the transfusion rate; this should never be too fast.
	• Observe for undue dyspnoea and frothy sputum.
Allergic reaction to blood	• Record temperature hourly.
	• Report any rise from base-line and any rigors.
	• Observe for any rashes.
Thrombophlebitis	• Handle infusion equipment only with clean, dry hands.
	• Remove bandage at least twice daily.
	• Report any swelling or redness of the cannula site. Change giving set every 24–48 hours.
Displacement of cannula	• Advise Miss Grange not to use her affected arm and hand.
	• Observe the cannula site for swelling and leakage.

7   The nurse should ensure that Miss Grange is aware of the need to continue with vitamin B_{12} injections (4–6 weekly) for the rest of her life. The community nurse will arrange these with her.

She should also be aware of the foods that are rich in iron such as liver, beef and green leafy vegetables to prevent a dietary deficiency anaemia.

1.2   Miss Webb—an elderly patient with dementia

Miss Ida Webb is a 82-year-old spinster who, before her admission to the psychogeriatric unit, lived on her own in a large Victorian house on the outskirts of the town. She has no known relatives.

She was admitted to hospital after she was found wandering about the town, unable to remember her address or her way home. A diagnosis of senile dementia has been made.

On investigation, her neighbours report that she has become gradually more incompetent. She has been found wandering in the garden at night and seems to have become dirty and unkempt recently. She has only become aggressive when they have offered help.

1   A junior colleague asks you to differentiate between confusion and dementia. How will you answer?

2   How will the degree of Miss Webb's mental state on admission be assessed?

3   How can the ward environment help to build up Miss Webb's sense of her own identity?

4   Explain how the nursing staff can avoid Miss Webb becoming aggressive.

5   How can Miss Webb be prevented from wandering?

6   Describe how the occupational therapist may assist in Miss Webb's care.

7   What arrangements can be made regarding Miss Webb's home? What happens to her pension?

8   One evening you find Miss Webb lying on the floor by her bed. She says that she fell. What actions should you take?

1.2 Answers

1 Ask your junior colleague to attempt a definition of both states (perhaps by comparing patients she has known). Then explain that confusion is usually abrupt in onset when it occurs in a previously well-orientated, independent person. The person suddenly becomes temporarily unable to understand his social and physical circumstances.

The most common cause of confusion is infection, but it may also be due to a change of environment, fluid and electrolyte imbalance, drugs, physical or psychological trauma, or cerebral anoxia.

Chronic brain failure (dementia) is characterized by permanent mental impairment due to loss of nerve cells from the brain. The onset is gradual and the person gradually loses his initiative, competence and memory, especially for recent events. This dementia becomes gradually worse, especially when the person is isolated from social contact by failure of sight or hearing, loneliness or physical handicap.

2 In order to assess the degree of Miss Webb's mental state, consider the following:

Mood Is she elated, irritable, anxious, withdrawn, suspicious, apathetic, agitated, aggressive?

Thought contact Does she experience any hallucinations, delusions or paranoid ideas?

Orientation Does she know who she is? where she is? where she lives? the date and day?

Insight Does she try to conceal gaps in her memory by fabrication? (confabulation)

---

3 • Address her by name.
 • Give her a name badge.
 • Name her locker and belongings.
 • Give her belongings that are hers alone.
 • Ensure that her bed is readily identifiable (e.g. by a coloured blanket).
 • Allow her to do as she pleases (providing it is safe).
 • Ensure that a clock and calender are easily observable to help her retain orientation.

- Plan a daily routine so that this regular daily framework helps her to remember.
- Encourage her to talk about her past achievements.

4
- Offer constant explanations, reminders and reassurances. (Mentally impaired people easily forget what they have been told.)
- Always be tactful and kind. Do not hurry her. (Miss Webb will be sensitive to the emotional atmosphere and will respond best to a calm, friendly environment.)

5   Miss Webb should not be locked in as patients such as this do not tend to make aggressive efforts to get through a door that will not open easily. An extra door handle above eye level will be sufficient to restrain her. Her bed should not be near a main exit.

However, the problem is best managed by ensuring that Miss Webb is kept occupied. She may be able to do odd tasks around the ward, e.g. arranging flowers, helping with bed-making.

Try and ascertain the cause for any restlessness. Such behaviour may be due to thirst, hunger, or a full bladder or bowel.

6   The occupational therapist can help to keep Miss Webb occupied. He/she can also help Miss Webb to regain her self-esteem by helping her to have a more constructive and productive life. Not only will the occupational therapist find interesting things for Miss Webb to do; he/she will also help to draw Miss Webb into group activities.

Craft work may help Miss Webb to gain a sense of achievement and accomplishment. This could be simple bead threading or tapestry work, depending on Miss Webb's interest and ability.

Music, quizzes or singing may be activities that Miss Webb may enjoy in a group. Domestic tasks such as bed-making or laying the table can also be done in pairs and may help to make Miss Webb feel worthwhile.

7   **Home** If Miss Webb has no relatives and will obviously not be fit enough to ever return home, her property will be put in the hands of a solicitor to be sold. The money will be kept in trust for her, but on her death, the money will revert to the state.

Pension When an elderly person is in hospital, his pension is reduced when he has been in hospital for more than 8 weeks. After a year in hospital it is reduced again. The medical social worker will usually take care of the person's pension book and the collection of the pension.

8   • Firstly check Miss Webb for injuries. Has she hit her head? Reassure her.
- If there seems to be no obvious injury, find another nurse to help you lift her back into bed.
- Try and ascertain from Miss Webb or any other witnesses exactly what happened. Determine and record Miss Webb's vital signs.
- Inform the doctor and nursing officer of the incident.
- Complete an accident form. Be sure to record only what *you know* to have happened. (Other patients or Miss Webb's account should be recorded as: 'The patient states that . . .') Note the time at which you informed the doctor and when he examined Miss Webb. Ask him to complete the incident form. If any X-rays are ordered, the results of these should also be recorded before the form is sent to the nursing office.
- Record the incident in the nursing record system.
- Reconsider Miss Webb's care plan. (In the light of this incident does it need to be modified? Why did the incident occur? Is there anything that could be done to prevent a reoccurrence?)

1.3   Mrs Parke—an elderly woman with cardiac failure

Mrs Emily Parke, aged 72 years, has been admitted to the ward with cardiac failure. On admission she is breathless and expectorating frothy sputum. She complains of increasing swelling of her ankles and lower legs, indigestion and constipation. She has also found it difficult to concentrate and remember things. She tires easily.

Mrs Parke lives in a terraced house in the middle of town. Her husband died 18 months ago. They had no family as Mrs Parke developed mitral stenosis following a bout of rheumatic fever when she was 18 years old.

1   What specific information will the nurse require from Mrs Parke on admission in order to plan her care?

2   What should be the initial aims or objectives of Mrs Parke's nursing care regarding the following problems:
   - Difficulty in breathing unless sitting upright in bed (respirations = 40 per minute)?
   - Expectoration of copious amounts of frothy sputum due to pulmonary oedema?
   - Poor appetite due to indigestion?
   - Constipation?
   - An inability to care for her own hygiene due to exhaustion?
   - Potential problems of immobility due to an inability to move freely in bed?
   - Discomfort of the legs and sacrum due to oedema?
   - Difficulty with concentration and memory due to cerebral anoxia?

3   With reference to altered anatomy and physiology explain Mrs Parke's symptoms to a junior colleague.

4   What nursing actions could be implemented to ensure Mrs Parke's rest and comfort?

Mrs Parke has been prescribed digoxin and frusemide by the doctor. A junior nurse on the ward plans to take her drug assessment later in the week.

5   What should the junior nurse know about Mrs Parke's drugs?

6   How can the nurse monitor the effect of Mrs Parke's medication?

In 3 weeks time Mrs Parke is much improved and ready for discharge.

---

7   How will the nurse evaluate Mrs Parke's care?

8   What community services will help Mrs Parke at home?

9   What advice can be given to Mrs Parke to help her remain in optimum health?

1.3   Answers

1
- **Breathlessness** Observe Mrs Parke's respirations at rest and on exertion. Ask her how it interferes with her normal activities. In what position is it less of a problem?
- **Cough and sputum** When is this a particular problem? Is the sputum difficult to cough up?
- **Indigestion** How does this manifest itself? Does she take anything to relieve it? What can she eat?
- **Constipation** What is her definition of this? What is her usual pattern of defecation? Does she take anything to relieve it?
- **Swelling of ankles** When is this worse? Does her abdomen feel swollen too? Observe the sacral area for oedema.
- **Impaired memory and concentration** How does this disturb her most? Does she have any way to help her remember?
- **Tiredness** How much does this interfere with her daily activities? Does she have a nap during the day?
- **Social history** How many stairs does she have to manage? Is her bathroom upstairs? How does she normally cope with housework and shopping?

2

Problems	Aims of care
Difficulty in breathing unless sitting upright in bed (respirations = 40 per minute)	For Mrs Parke to breathe more easily
Expectoration of copious amounts of frothy sputum due to pulmonary oedema	For Mrs Parke to be able to expectorate
Poor appetite due to indigestion	For Mrs Parke to be able to eat without discomfort
Constipation	For Mrs Parke to open her bowels in her usual pattern
Inability to care for her own hygiene due to exhaustion	For Mrs Parke to feel clean, rested and comfortable

Potential problems of immobility due to an inability to move freely in bed	For Mrs Parke's skin to remain intact For Mrs Parke's peripheral and respiratory circulation to be maintained
Discomfort of the legs and sacrum due to oedema	For Mrs Parke not to be troubled by her oedematous areas
Difficulty with concentration and memory due to cerebral anoxia	For Mrs Parke to feel that her mental powers have improved

3

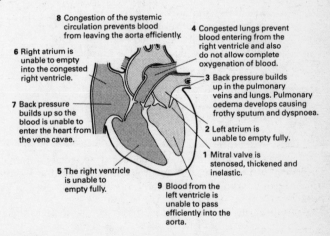

Fig. 2 Complications arising from cardiac failure.

Congested lungs cause poor oxygenation of circulating blood. Low oxygen content of blood means poor function of major organs; cerebral anoxia leads to tiredness and memory and concentration impairment. Hypoxia of the portal circulation results in poor digestion, leading to dyspepsia and constipation. Congestion of the systemic circulation causes fluid to build up in dependent tissues.

4
- Keep her in an upright position either with pillows or a back rest in bed or in a chair.
- Provide her with sedatives if necessary to help her to rest.

- Provide reassurance and support and be readily available as breathlessness may be very frightening.
- Plan care to incorporate rest periods.
- Help with change of position 2-hourly and provide sheepskins to prevent soreness resulting from immobility.

5 **Digoxin** slows the heart rate and strengthens its beat. These two actions help the weakened heart to pump blood more efficiently. It enables the ventricles to empty more completely after each systolic contraction and reduces the size of the heart during diastole. (A smaller, stronger heart pumps more efficiently than a large, flabby one.)

Relatively large doses are given initially so that therapeutic levels accumulate. A small daily maintenance dose can then be given. It is possible to over-digitalize, especially in elderly patients, so it is important to check the apical pulse before administering the drug. It is not usually given if the pulse falls below 60 beats/min. Other signs of digoxin toxicity are dropped beats, a coupled pulse, and nausea and vomiting.

Frusemide is given to rid the body of excess fluid and sodium that has built up in the tissues. It acts on the tubules of the nephron to inhibit tubular reabsorption, resulting in increased diuresis.

The loss of sodium causes the kidney to also secrete excess potassium, so it is important to observe the patient for signs of potassium depletion (hypokalaemia). Weak pulse, hypotension and generalized weakness are features of low potassium. A potassium supplement is always given with frusemide to minimize this side-effect.

The increased diuresis can be exhausting at first so Mrs Parke should be lifted onto the commode.

6 **Digoxin**
- Take 4-hourly apex-radial recordings.
- Note any slowing of the apex–radial beat below 60 beats/min. Inform the doctor before administration if such a bradycardia is present.
- Report any irregularity of the beat.

Frusemide
- Weigh daily every morning before breakfast ensuring that Mrs Parke is wearing similar clothing each day.
- Measure the intake and output to monitor the degree of diuresis and prevent dehydration.
- Make a visual assessment of the degree of oedema.

7 Relate to your initial aims of care.

Difficulty in breathing
- Is Mrs Parke less breathless? Can she move around without undue dyspnoea? Are her respirations less than 40 per minute?

Expectoration of frothy sputum
- Has this ceased or become minimal?

Poor appetite
- Is Mrs Parke able to eat without indigestion?

Constipation
- Have Mrs Parke's bowel habits returned to normal?

Inability to care for her own hygiene
- Was her hygiene maintained to her satisfaction?
- Has this problem ceased?

Potential problems of immobility
- Has her skin remained intact?
- Have there been any problems relating to chest infection or thrombosis/embolus?
- Will she be able to manage mobility at home?

Discomfort of the legs and sacrum due to oedema
- Was her comfort maintained?
- Is the oedema less marked?

Difficulty with concentration and memory
- Does Mrs Parke think this is better?
- Is she safe to care for herself?

8   The services needed by Mrs Parke will depend on her condition on discharge. Possible support services are:
- Meals on Wheels—to provide a cooked mid-day meal.
- Home help—to do heavy housework and shopping.
- Geriatric day hospital—to provide company as well as a midday meal and also to provide a regular means of reassessment by nursing staff.
- Community nurse—to check her condition and help her in the bath if necessary.
- Luncheon club—to provide company and cooked midday meal and sometimes to provide afternoon entertainment.

9   If Mrs Parke still has problems with memory and concentration, the following advice must also be written down:
- Report any recurrence of breathlessness on exertion, unusual fatigue or weakness, swelling of ankles, or frothy sputum.
- Report any nausea and vomiting, or palpitations.

- Take activity as you feel able but have a rest during the day.
- Sleep may be easier if supported by three or four pillows.
- Always take tablets as prescribed.
- It is advisable not to smoke, eat large 'heavy' meals, or drink alcohol in excess.
- Avoid a high dietary salt intake. Do not add salt to food at the table and try to exclude crisps, nuts, salty meats and bacon.

1.4 Mrs Betts—an elderly woman with hypothermia

Mrs Cynthia Betts, a 72-year-old widow, lives alone in a terraced house. One winter morning she slipped on the way to her dustbin. Some hours later she was found by her neighbour whom she did not recognize. She is now to be admitted to the acute geriatric ward in a state of semiconsciousness and hypothermia. Her temperature on admission was 32°C.

1 Explain how a junior colleague could be helped to prepare for Mrs Betts' admission into the ward.
2 Identify Mrs Betts' actual problems on admission.
3 Stating aims, plan the care that should be implemented to overcome the above problems. Give reasons for all actions.
4 Describe how Mrs Betts' risk of developing pressure areas may be assessed.

Mrs Betts gradually regains consciousness and her temperature returns to normal. By the third day after admission she is able to get out of bed and is eating and drinking normally.

5 As soon as Mrs Betts regained consciousness she began to become agitated about her cat, Tibbles. How can she be reassured?
6 Outline a suitable diet for Mrs Betts, justifying the choice with reference to the principles of a balanced diet.
7 What are the responsibilities of the nurse-in-charge at meal-times in Mrs Betts' ward?

When Mrs Betts is ready for discharge her son, who lives 100 miles away, visits. He says his mother should move into a home as she is lonely and her house is too big and cold for her. Mrs Betts is adamant that she wants to stay at home and that she is quite mobile and independent. At the next weekly case conference Mrs Betts' case is discussed. In view of her feelings and also her abilities it is decided to let her return home and to monitor her progress.

8   Explain the use of case conferences in the care of the elderly.
9   Describe the advice Mrs Betts should be given on discharge to avoid hypothermia indoors and outdoors.
10 Explain which one of the following would be most appropriate for Mrs Betts on discharge:
   (a) Home help
   (b) Luncheon club
   (c) Day hospital
   (d) Community nurse

1.4 Answers

1 Check the junior nurse's knowledge of hypothermia and its management. Mrs Betts will have a temperature of below 35°C. This will have caused a low metabolic rate resulting in low vital signs and an altered level of consciousness.

Then ask the junior colleague what she thinks will be necessary to prepare for Mrs Betts' admission. As she prepares each item an explanation can be given, thus:

- **Warm cubicle** This provides a warm environment, ideally about 28°C (80°F).
- **Space blanket** This insulates the patient and prevents further heat loss.
- **Low reading rectal thermometer (or rectal probe)** Rectal temperatures reflect the deep body temperature.
- **Emergency equipment (suction, oxygen, intravenous infusion stand)** This provides a means of maintaining a clear airway and a means of correcting a fluid and electrolyte imbalance. (A cardiac monitor may be used to monitor the cardiac rhythm.)
- **Sheepskin ripple bed** Mrs Betts, because of her semiconscious state and poor condition, will be immobile and at risk of developing pressure sores.

2
- Low temperature
- Depressed circulatory/respiratory systems ⎱ resulting
- Altered level of consciousness ⎰ from the low temperature

- Dehydration
- Possibly other injuries due to the fall

3

Problem	Aim	Care	Rationale
Low temperature	To raise the body temperature by 0.5°C hourly	• Nurse in a side ward • Use a fan heater to heat room to 28°C. • Wrap patient in a space blanket (shiny side next to patient). • Monitor patient's rectal temperature half-hourly.	If the temperature is raised too quickly the patient will experience a sudden increase in metabolic rate, and circulatory failure may develop when the heart cannot cope with this extra demand.

Unable to maintain own airway due to altered level of consciousness	To maintain a clear airway	• Position in recovery position. • Keep suction and oxygen at hand.	Semiconscious patients may asphyxiate due to the tongue falling back and occluding the airway, or the aspiration of vomit or secretions.
Depressed respirations	To increase oxygenation	Give oxygen via a ventimask 38% at 4 litres per minute as prescribed.	If oxygen is not replaced respiratory failure may result.
Bradycardia and hypotension	To monitor the circulatory system	• Observe the cardiac rhythm on an oscilloscope. • Check and record pulse and blood pressure half-hourly. • Report any further reduction in blood pressure or pulse rate and irregularity of pulse.	Dysrhythmias are a common cause of death in hypothermia. Any further deterioration in vital signs may mean re-warming is too fast.
Dehydration	To replace fluid without overloading the circulation	Give intravenous fluids as prescribed.	Dehydration will cause further lowering of the blood pressure and electrolyte imbalance. A failing heart may not be able to cope with a sudden increase in circulating fluids.

Potential other injuries	To observe the patient for any other effects of her fall	Observe the patient for bruises, cuts and any other deformity of the limbs.	If other injuries are not treated, the patient may deteriorate.

4   Mrs Betts' risk of developing pressure sores may be assessed using the Norton score (devised by Norton et al., 1962).

Her condition will be assessed on the five categories as below:

Physical condition		Mental condition		Activity		Mobility		Incontinence	
Good	4	Alert	4	Ambulant	4	Full	4	None	4
Fair	3	Apathetic	3	Slightly limited	3	Slightly limited	3	Occasionally	3
Poor	2	Confused	2	Very limited	2	Very limited	2	Usually of urine	2
Very bad	1	Stuporous	1	Bedfast	1	Immobile	1	Of urine and faeces	1

If a patient scores a total of 14 or below, he is considered 'at risk' of developing pressure sores.

Mrs Betts would probably score 5–7 so she is obviously very much at risk.

5   Inform the medical social worker who will arrange for the house to be checked to ensure that it is safe (e.g. no fires/gas left on). She will either arrange for a willing neighbour to feed Tibbles or arrange temporary care by the RSPCA.

6   Obviously there is a wide range of suitable diets that could be chosen, but you need to give reasons for *your* choice which relate to the elderly *and* to the principles of a well-balanced diet.

The diet of an elderly person should be high in vitamins, proteins and minerals as the elderly have diminished absorption of nutrients.

There should be sufficient calories for the maintenance of

energy and activity, but as metabolism is slower, approximately 1500 calories per day are needed.

In the elderly there is less mobility and a diminished intestinal lubrication which predisposes to constipation. Thus, added dietary fibre and an adequate fluid intake (2–3 litres per day) is important. Fluids are also important to eliminate metabolic waste as kidney function is less efficient.

Meals should be small and easily digestible. An elderly person is often less active and finds it difficult to digest large, 'heavy' meals.

7
- Patients are taken to the toilet before meal-times.
- Ambulant patients are seated around the dining table to make meal-times a social event, if they wish.
- Non-ambulant patients are in a suitable position for eating.
- Each individual patient is served according to the state of his dentures, his likes and dislikes regarding food and fluids, his preference for a cooked meal at midday or evening or both, his normal bowel habit, and any special diets.
- Hot food is kept hot.
- Portions are small and attractively served.
- Alternatives ('Build-up', egg dishes, sandwiches) are offered if the meal is not wanted.
- Help is given when necessary (adapted cutlery, food cut up or help with feeding).
- Non slip mats and serviettes are used to avoid spillage.
- Staff evaluate if their patients have eaten well and find out the reasons for not eating.

8
The care of the elderly is multidisciplinary and depends on good teamwork between the different disciplines involved.

Good teamwork depends on good communication and liaison. Therefore, case conferences are held on a regular basis to discuss patients' progress and discharge plans. Personnel involved in the case conference will be the patient's doctor, primary nurse, physiotherapist, occupational therapist, social worker and community nurse.

Ideally, the conference team assesses the patient's progress in their individual fields and considers any problems that may arise on discharge. In this way, domestic problems can be overcome before discharge and the patient can be discharged safely as soon as he is ready. Community services will have already been notified and can ensure that care is continued as necessary.

In theory, research seems to indicate that the ideal is not happening and that patients are sent home unprepared [Skeet Muriel (1970) *Home from Hospital*. London: The Dan Mason Nursing Research Committee].

9   **Indoors** The medical social worker can assess the heating. Mrs Betts will probably be entitled to a grant for roof insulation and help with her heating bills.

In winter she should wear extra clothing, especially at night, and try to stay in one room which she can heat well. Any draughts under doors should be stopped with cushions or newspaper.

Outdoors Mrs Betts should be advised to wrap up warmly, particularly ensuring that her head, hands and feet are well covered.

In the winter she should move her dustbin close to the back door and put salt down to melt any ice.

10   (b) is the *most* appropriate as Mrs Betts is now healthy, mobile, independent and able to care for herself. However, she is lonely and a luncheon club would provide the stimulation of others' company and group involvement, as well as providing a meal.

1.5   Mr Green—an elderly man with osteoarthrosis

Mr Albert Green, aged 78 years, lives in a ground floor flat in a sheltered housing scheme. He has suffered increasing disability, due to osteoarthrosis of his hips and knees, and poor vision. However, until recently he had been able to maintain his independence and to walk short distances with a walking frame.

Mrs Green died suddenly last month following a stroke. Since then, Mr Green has become more withdrawn and immobile. The warden rang the general practitioner when he found Mr Green lying in bed saying he wanted to die and refusing to eat or move. The general practitioner referred Mr Green to the community nursing services.

1   Discuss the benefits of sheltered housing schemes.
2   How may the community nurse explain the effects of osteoarthrosis to the student nurse accompanying her?
3   Describe the other physical effects of ageing that Mr Green may display.
4   What support can the community nurse offer to Mr Green in this period of bereavement?

Gradually Mr Green overcame his apathy and began to continue his usual activities. However, his period of immobility had left him stiff and less active.

His general practitioner has revised his drug therapy and has prescribed:

benorylate	10 ml 4-hourly as required
indomethacin	25 mg 8-hourly
multivitamins	2 tablets daily
imipramine	10 mg 8-hourly

Mr Green admits that he has problems taking his drugs at the correct time as his wife had always looked after them for him.

5   How can Mr Green be helped to regain his mobility?
6   What aids can be given to Mr Green to help him maintain his independence?
7   State the problems an elderly patient may experience which may make compliance with drug therapy difficult.

8   How can Mr Green be helped to take his medications as prescribed?
9   In what way is each drug effective and what advice should Mr Green be given about his drugs?
10 What continuing community support can be offered to Mr Green now that he is no longer in need of nursing care?

1.5   Answers

1   Sheltered housing schemes consist of approximately thirty
units (bungalows, two-storey flats and one-bedroomed flat-
lets) all connected to a warden by an audio alarm.

The benefits of such schemes are that the housing is
specifically designed for the needs of the elderly so that
they provide an immediate means of help in an emergency,
and give elderly people the company of others.

The major disadvantage occurs if the residents become
ill. The warden may then have to take on an extended role
for which he or she has not been trained.

2   The community nurse may ask the learner nurse what she
knows about osteoarthrosis. She can then expand on the
student's present knowledge. She will need to explain that
osteoarthrosis is a form of degenerative joint disease which
is probably present to some degree in all elderly people.

Ageing and wear and tear gradually destroys the articulating cartilage covering the joints. Flakes of cartilage lie loose
in the joints and sometimes harden and clarify to form 'loose
bodies' which restrain movement in the affected joints. The
bones that make up the joint also become hardened and
cysts may develop. At the edges of joints, bony growths
('osteophytes' or 'spurs') develop, causing a gnarled and
knobbly appearance.

Diagrams (see Fig. 3) are useful to illustrate the explanation.

3   Physical changes that may have been noticeable in Mr Green
due to the ageing process are:

Height reduction Shortening of the vertebrae and thinning of the
intervertebral discs results in an average reduction in height of
2 inches.

Loss of mobility Muscle fibres atrophy with age and are replaced by
fibrous tissue, resulting in swelling of the joints and fusion of
articulating cartilages. These changes result in loss of mobility and
agility.

Appearance Loss of tissue elasticity causes a dry, wrinkled appearance.
Loss of subcutaneous fat may add to the wizened effect. Body hair
regresses with age, which may cause thinning or baldness.

Sight After the age of 10 years the lens gradually loses its elasticity.
Thus, the inability to focus clearly on near objects (presbyopia) is
common in the elderly.

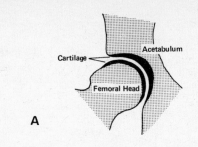

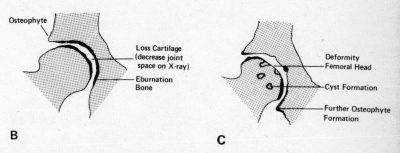

Fig. 3 Osteoarthrosis of the hip.

Hearing By the age of 60 years most people have lost 75% of their ability to hear high frequency sounds. This is due to a combination of increased cerumen, rigidity of the ossicles, and atrophy of the auditory nerve.

4   The nurse should recognize that the first phase of mourning usually results in the bereaved person needing to talk about the deceased. She should provide a compassionate atmosphere and be a good listener. She should reassure Mr Green that crying, loss of appetite, inability to sleep and lack of concentration are common features of bereavement and that he should not feel inadequate because of these symptoms.

She should try to help Mr Green to feel that his life is still worthwhile. Involvement with outside agencies (e.g. Cruse—the national organization for the widowed and their children) may help him to come to terms with the loss of his wife.

5   It is important to ensure that Mr Green's pain is under control before attempting to remobilize him.

His limbs should be put through a full range of movements to overcome their stiffness before he attempts to walk. He should sit with his feet up to straighten his knees and lie prone on some nights to straighten his hips.

A community physiotherapist may be available to help. A place at the geriatric day hospital may provide physiotherapy and heat treatment, and may also give skilled counselling for his bereavement.

6   Osteoarthrosis of the hips and knees causes particular problems in getting up to a standing position and bending down. Useful aids may therefore include:
   • raised toilet seat
   • high-seated chair (or a self-lift chair)
   • bath bridge
   • long-handled shoe horn
   • stocking aid (to put on socks)
   • monkey pole over the bed

7   • Not understanding, remembering or hearing properly initial directions from the doctor
   • Inability to read instructions on the label of medicine bottles
   • Forgetfulness, which may result in dosages being missed or taken twice
   • Inability to open 'child-proof' containers
   • Large tablets, which may be difficult to swallow
   • Side-effects or no immediate effect, may result in the person discontinuing the drug of his own accord

8   • The chemist must be asked to dispense Mr Green's medications in easy-to-open, large containers.
   • Larger instruction labels can be affixed and each different medication colour-coded to facilitate recognition.
   • A large, colour-coded chart can be put on the wall as a reminder of daily dosages.
   • Putting the day's tablets in separate dispensers marked with the appropriate time would help to prevent missing doses or repeating them.

9   Benorylate is to relieve his pain and 10 ml may be taken whenever he has pain. However, he should not repeat this within 4 hours.

Indomethacin is to reduce the inflammation in his joints and will also reduce the pain. It must be taken regularly, three times a day. It can cause sickness if taken on an empty stomach, so it should be taken after a meal or with a milky drink.

Multivitamins are tablets containing a mixture of vitamins to maintain one's general health. He is to take two tablets once a day. The time at which he takes these is not important.

Imipramine is to help reduce his depression. He must take one of these three times a day. He should not expect a dramatic improvement as they will take about a fortnight to take effect.

10 A home help will undertake any domestic tasks normally performed by Mrs Green and which Mr Green will be unable to do because of his immobility.

A day centre will provide exercise to help Mr Green achieve maximum mobility. It will also provide a cooked lunch as Mr Green may not have the ability or the desire to cook or eat by himself. Day centres can also provide chiropody— Mr Green will be unable to care for his own feet because of his stiff hips.

The general practitioner or health visitor for the elderly can visit Mr Green at 4–6-hourly intervals to monitor his condition.

1.6   Mrs Hopkirk—an elderly woman with Parkinson's disease

Mrs Hilda Hopkirk, is aged 80 years, admitted for a period of physiotherapy/occupational therapy and control of her drug therapy.

Mrs Hopkirk has lived with her daughter and son-in-law and two teenage grandchildren since Mr Hopkirk's death 10 years ago. Until recently she has been quite mobile and independent. However, in the last few months she has become bed-bound with periods of mild confusion. Her general practitioner has diagnosed Parkinson's disease and advised admission to hospital.

On admission she is immobile and seems withdrawn and depressed. Her speech is difficult to understand and her daughter says she eats very little and has lost 8kg in weight.

1   Explain to a junior colleague the reasons for Mrs Hopkirk's problems.
2   Using a problem-solving approach plan nursing actions to help overcome Mrs Hopkirk's problems on admission.
3   Describe how the above care can be evaluated.
4   Mrs Hopkirk's confusion becomes particularly apparent at night. List, giving reasons, the actions that may be taken to overcome this.
5   Mrs Hopkirk is incontinent of urine at times. Discuss the possible reasons for this.

Mrs Hopkirk is prescribed Sinemet. She has daily physiotherapy and begins to walk slowly with a frame. She also attends the occupational therapy department daily and is becoming more independent and happier.

6   Describe the nursing care Mrs Hopkirk will need in relation to the potential side-effects of her drug therapy.
7   While you are in charge of the ward, Mrs Hopkirk's daughter complains to you that her mother has not been bathed since her admission. How will you manage this complaint?
8   What advice and support may be offered to Mrs Hopkirk and her daughter before discharge?

1.6 Answers

1 In Parkinson's disease there is degeneration of the basal
   ganglia (an area of grey matter within the inner cortex of
   the brain). This portion of the brain produces dopamine, a
   chemical transmitter which is essential for smooth motor
   activities. Therefore, parkinsonism results in depletion of
   dopamine and the patient experiences difficulty with all
   types of muscular movement. This is shown by tremor,
   rigidity and, eventually, immobility.

   Rigidity of the facial muscles causes the patient to have
   difficulty in chewing and swallowing. These problems with
   eating, together with the embarrassment of such problems,
   often mean that the patient eats little and loses weight.

   The patient can also become very depressed by his
   inability to maintain his independence.

2

Problem	Aim	Action
Immobility (due to rigidity of muscles)	To help Mrs Hopkirk to initiate movement	• Rock Mrs Hopkirk back and forth before any movement. • Teach Mrs Hopkirk to imagine an obstacle to be overcome by parts of her body that she wants to move. • Plan daily physiotherapy.
	To help to prevent the following complications of immobility: pressure sores	• Help Mrs Hopkirk to change her position 2–4-hourly.
	contractures thromboembolism	• Encourage limb movements and deep breathing.
	constipation	• Encourage 2 litres of fluid daily.

Withdrawn and depressed	To promote independence and self-esteem	• Let Mrs Hopkirk do as much for herself as possible. • Call the patient by her name if she requests. • Let the patient wear her own clothes.
	To find out the reason(s) for these feelings	• Encourage Mrs Hopkirk to talk about her feelings.
Difficulty in communication	To help Mrs Hopkirk to communicate clearly	• Show Mrs Hopkirk how to exaggerate her lip movements. • Give the patient time to express herself.
Weight loss (due to difficulty in chewing and swallowing)	To maintain adequate nutrition	• Provide her with a high calorie/high protein, soft diet. • Give small frequent meals (so the meals are always hot). • Provide straws for drinking. • Plan a rest period before meals. • Provide favourite foods.

3
- **Immobility** Increased mobility will not be measurable in a day. Staff relatives and the patient herself should notice improvement at the end of a week. Progress should be reported as to her steadiness and the degree of movement achieved. Have the suggested actions helped Mrs Hopkirk to move?

  Potential complications should be assessed daily by noting the colour and state of Mrs Hopkirk's skin over pressure areas, any stiffness or malposition of her limbs, any redness of her calves, and her bowel movements if they are not within normal patterns.
- **Withdrawn and depressed** A daily evaluation is probably not realistic but any increased depression must be noted so that nursing care can be reconsidered.

Any conversation with Mrs Hopkirk that helps to reveal further causes for her depression should obviously be noted.

At the end of a week Mrs Hopkirk should be asked if she feels any happier.

- **Difficulty in communication** Note on a weekly basis if communication is becoming clearer. A daily progress report can be made on how Mrs Hopkirk is managing her speech exercises. Check with relatives and the physiotherapist about improvement in speech.
- **Weight loss** Mrs Hopkirk should only be weighed weekly but a daily assessment can be made on how much she is managing to eat.

4
- One nurse should be primarily responsible for Mrs Hopkirk at night. New faces will only add to her confusion.
- The assigned nurse should explain all care carried out and remind the patient of her location and reason for hospitalization, to reinforce self-identity.
- Mrs Hopkirk's usual night routine should be adhered to as far as possible. Continuity with her usual lifestyle will prevent further confusion.
- A shaded light should be left at bedside as darkness in an unfamiliar environment will add to confusion.
- Mrs Hopkirk should not be sedated as sedation frequently exacerbates confusion.

5
- In an unfamiliar environment Mrs Hopkirk may find it difficult to find the toilet or lack of mobility may make it difficult for her to reach the toilet.
- She may not like to ask the assistance of the nurses or know how to call them.
- She may feel so depressed that she cannot be bothered about continence.
- She may have a urinary infection, especially if incontinence is a long-standing problem.
- Uterine displacement or faecal impaction may be local causes of incontinence.

6

Potential side-effect of Sinemet	Related nursing care
Gastrointestinal disorders (anorexia, nausea and vomiting)	Give the drug with food, in the middle of a meal.

Hypotension	Take daily blood pressure recordings and report any recording of diastolic pressure lower than the base-line reading.
Psychological abnormalities (depression, paranoia)	Observe the patient for hostility, lowering of mood, and delusions.
Cardiac arrhythmias	Record the pulse 4-hourly and report any irregularities in its rate or rhythm.

7   • Stay calm and polite. Invite Mrs Hopkirk's daughter into Sister's office (or another quiet, private place) to discuss her complaint.
    • Ask why she thinks her mother has not been bathed.
    • Respect her judgement if her answer is at all likely. Promise you will investigate and give her a definite time to discuss the results of your findings.
    • If you cannot defuse the situation, call the nursing officer (who must be informed of the incident at some stage anyway).
    • Make a report of the incident. In Sister's absence, begin to investigate the complaint. Check Mrs Hopkirk's care plan for mention of hygiene care and find out who has cared for her since her admission.

8   **Advice** Remind Mrs Hopkirk and her daughter that Sinemet should be taken in the middle of meals to avoid gastric upsets.

Constipation is a common problem in patients with Parkinson's disease. Mrs Hopkirk should try to have a daily walk, eat roughage in her diet and drink about 5 pints of liquid a day.

Remind both women of the actions in Mrs Hopkirk's care plan that have proved effective in minimizing her problems.

Support Twice weekly (or more) visits to the day hospital will relieve Mrs Hopkirk's daughter and provide continued physiotherapy, occupational therapy and speech therapy for her mother.

Aids, such as a commode, could be lent to the family if Mrs Hopkirk has problems in reaching the toilet.

2 Care of the Patient with a Sensory Impairment

2.1   Mrs Summers—a blind adult in hospital

Mrs Summers is 38 years old and has been blind since birth. She is married with two children aged 10 and 12 years. Mrs Summers has had a guide dog for about 10 years and is a part-time telephonist in a local college.

Mrs Summers has been admitted to the ward for minor surgery and expects to be in hospital for about 4 days. Her husband is having time off work in order to look after the children and the dog.

1   What information should the nurse ascertain during the admission interview in order to maintain Mrs Summers' normal level of independence during her stay?

2   What important actions should the nurse take on admission to orientate Mrs Summers to the ward?

3   What would you tell a junior nurse about communicating with Mrs Summers?

4   How can the nurse ensure that meal-times are a pleasurable experience for Mrs Summers?

5   What actions should the nurse take to ensure Mrs Summers' safety during hospitalization?

6   As nurse in charge of the ward, what would be your response if Mrs Summers asks if her husband can bring in the dog to see her?

Mrs Summers recovers well after her operation and is up and about the following day.

7   How can Mrs Summers be occupied during her convalescent period before being discharged home?

8   What facilities are available in the community to help Mrs Summers maintain her independence?

2.1 Answers

1

Mobility
- Does she use a long cane to move about with when she does not have the dog?
- How does she orientate herself to a new environment?
- How does she like to be helped when moving around?

Hygiene needs
- How much help does she need in meeting her hygiene needs? Does she use showers or baths?

Dressing
- How can the nurse help when it comes to choosing what clothes to wear? Does she have a means of identifying various articles of clothing?
- Does she need any help with applying make-up and doing her hair?
- How can the nurse arrange her belongings so that she can find them herself?

Eating and drinking
- What are her likes and dislikes?
- How does she like her food to be served?
- Does she need any help with eating?

Miscellaneous
- Is there anything else that the nursing staff need to know in order for her to maintain her independence?

2
- Allow Mrs Summers to explore the environment with the guidance of a nurse, particularly:
  1 the area around her bed, call bell, radio, locker
  2 the bathroom and toilets
  3 the day room
- Orientate Mrs Summers to the fire exits.
- Introduce her to the staff who will be caring for her.
- Introduce her to the patients on either side of her.
- Show her where she can find the telephone.

3
- When speaking to Mrs Summers always address her by name so that she knows you are talking to her.
- Always introduce yourself so that she knows who she is talking to.
- Always tell her what you are going to do before you do

it, e.g. tell her that you are going to make her bed, give her a cup of tea, etc.

- At the end of a conversation always indicate that you are moving away—talking to nobody is embarrassing!
- Always address questions to Mrs Summers, never to people who are with her.
- Do not shout when talking to Mrs Summers—she is not deaf.

4
- Orientate Mrs Summers to the dining area so that she can join other patients for meals.
- Describe the meal to Mrs Summers and the position of different foods on the plate.
- Do not attempt to cut up the food for her. She may indicate a need for help with some foods, e.g. fish that has a lot of bones.
- Do not overfill cups or glasses and always tell her where the cup/glass is in relation to her plate.

5
- Ensure that there are no trailing flexes from equipment.
- Always clear up spillages immediately.
- Do not leave hot drinks where Mrs Summers might accidentally knock them over.
- Do not leave medicines on her locker top.
- Do not move articles of furniture around without telling her.

6   Mrs Summers' dog is obviously very important to her and is usually always with her. It is therefore reasonable that Mrs Summers should be allowed to see him while she is in hospital.

It is probably best that Mr Summers take the dog to the day room rather than bring him into the ward. Inform the hospital receptionist that Mr Summers is bringing in a 'guide dog'.

7
- Find out what she likes to do in her spare time.
- Provide her with talking books.
- Ensure that a radio/television is available for her use.
- Provide her with braille books/periodicals.
- Provide her with specially adapted games for the blind, e.g. chess, dominoes, Scrabble.

8
- A guide dog—from the Guide Dogs for the Blind Association
- Facilities from the Royal National Institute for the Blind
- The British Talking Book Service
- Concessions to blind persons from British Rail
- Day Centres/social clubs available through the welfare services

- Financial assistance—special income tax allowance
- Writing aids—to write letters in braille
- Braille wrist watches and alarm clocks
- Aids for the house for cooking and measuring ingredients (including controls for gas and electric cookers)

2.2   Mrs Wilson—an elderly lady with cataracts

Mrs Ada Wilson, aged 72 years, has bilateral cataracts and has been admitted to the ward for surgery to the left eye. Mrs Wilson lives on her own but is very active and often spends time with her married sons. Her sight has gradually been deteriorating over the past few years and she is now unable to cope without help.

1   Describe the care Mrs Wilson will require on admission to the ward in order for her to settle as quickly as possible.
2   With reference to normal and altered physiology how would you explain Mrs Wilson's condition to a junior nurse?
3   Outline the specific pre-operative management Mrs Wilson will require.

Mrs Wilson goes to theatre the day after admission for intracapsular extraction of the left lens.

4   Describe, giving reasons, the specific care Mrs Wilson will need post-operatively.
5   State the specific post-operative observations the nurse should make and explain their significance.
6   What should Mrs Wilson be taught about the instillation of eye drops in preparation for her discharge home?
7   What preparations should be made for her discharge and what other information/advice will she need?
8   Outline the different methods available for correcting Mrs Wilson's resultant loss of lens.

2.2 Answers

1 Mrs Wilson may have been able to move about easily at home despite her decreased vision, but hospital is an unfamiliar environment. It will be important to assess the degree of her sight defect and then to orientate her accordingly by:
   - orientating her to her bed and the essential items around it, e.g. call bell, radio, locker
   - introducing her to the nurses who will be looking after her.
   - showing her where the bathroom/toilets/day room are. Walk with her initially to point out any 'hazards' on the way and ensure that her bed is close to these areas.
   - introducing Mrs Wilson to the patients on either side of her
   - explaining visiting times for relatives

2 You should first define cataracts to the nurse [opacity (clouding) of the lens of the eye].
   In order to understand the altered physiology the junior nurse needs to understand the normal physiology of the eye. A diagram should be drawn to illustrate the anatomical position of the lens. The lens is a transparent, jelly-like structure which has the ability to change shape. The purpose of the lens is to:
   1 allow the transmission of light and visual images to reach the retina
   2 bring visual images into focus on the retina by altering its shape, i.e. 'accommodation'.
   The cause of 'senile cataracts' is unknown, but the opacity of the usually transparent lens occurs as a result of chemical changes in the protein of which the lens is made. The transmission of light rays is interrupted, resulting in blurred images. The lens swells and loses its ability to change shape. Accommodation is lost and objects become distorted and out of focus.

3 - An explanation of the operation and what it entails should be given (will probably be under local anaesthetic).
   - It should be explained to Mrs Wilson that she will not be able to focus at all with the left eye as the lens has been removed.
   - Eye swabs may be taken to rule out infection.
   - Eyes will be examined by the ophthalmologist to rule out infection.

- Eyelashes may be clipped to make access to the eye easier and to reduce the risk of infection.
- Mydriatic eye drops should be instilled as per prescription to dilate the pupil. Access to the lens is via the pupil.

4

Nursing care	Rationale
Mrs Wilson may be kept on bed rest for up to 24 hours with the head of the bed and one pillow elevated slightly. Mrs Wilson should move her head gently.	This prevents rapid pressure build-up within the eye which may exert stress on the suture line.
She should lie either on her back or on the unoperated side for a week post-operatively.	This reduces the danger of damage to the eye.
Change Mrs Wilson's dressing on the first post-operative day and daily thereafter. Eye drops should be instilled after cleansing and a sterile pad and/or Cartella shield placed over the eye.	Eyedrops will consist of a mydriatic (to dilate the pupil) and antibiotics. The eye is covered as protection against infection and pressure.
Observe for severe pain.	This could be indicative of intraocular haemorrhage.
Mrs Wilson may mobilize on the following day but she should: • move slowly • avoid bending over • control sneezing/coughing	Any sudden movement may increase intraocular pressure and cause haemorrhage.
Administer antiemetics as prescribed.	This prevents vomiting and head movement in order to decrease the risk of raised intraocular pressure.
Avoid any sudden movement or light.	This stimulates the patient to 'squeeze' eyes which can cause raised intraocular pressure.

5 • Note the shape of the pupil. It should be round and central and the degree of dilatation should be noted. Any

deviation must be reported as there is the possibility of a prolapsed iris.

- Report any pain as this could be indicative of iris prolapse or intraocular haemorrhage.
- Observe for photophobia, a red eye, a small pupil and a muddy iris, which would be indicative of post-operative iritis.

6 Mrs Wilson will need help to instil the eye drops. She may be able to get her family to help, so they should all be given the following instructions:

- Hands should be clean—wash before and after instillation.
- If the eye needs cleansing use sterile water and gauze/lint. Cotton wool must not be used as small fibres of cotton wool may become detached and remain in the eye.
- The lower lid should be pulled down. Mrs Williams should look up while eye drops are placed in the centre of the inside of the lower lid.
- The dropper must never touch the eye.
- The eyes should be closed slowly to avoid expulsion of the drops.
- Eye drops must be stored correctly.

7 - Order eye drops for her discharge.
- Arrange for the district nurse to visit Mrs Wilson after she has been discharged.
- Make an outpatient's appointment and arrange hospital transport if needed.
- Send a letter to Mrs Wilson's general practitioner.
- Ensure that Mrs Wilson has help to cope with any tasks that involve lifting/bending down.
- Instruct Mrs Wilson to wear her own glasses with the left lens shielded to minimize light to the newly operated eye. Full exposure to the light may cause discomfort.
- Advise her to wear the eye shield at night to avoid inadvertent rubbing.
- Inform her as to when the other eye will be treated.

8 - **Intraocular lens inplant** This would be carried out at the time of operation. It may cause an inflammatory reaction in the eye.
- **Contact lenses** These may be difficult for Mrs Wilson to manage.
- **Spectacles** These are good for the elderly. Mrs Wilson will need two pairs—one for near vision and one for distant vision.

2.3   Mr Bowen—a deaf man in hospital

Mr Bowen is 36 years old and has been admitted to the ward for an investigation of epigastric pain.

Mr Bowen has been deaf due to the effects of meningitis since he was 10 years old. During this infection the auditory nerves were damaged causing perceptive (sensori-neural) deafness.

Mr Bowen is married and has a 6-month old daughter. He is an architect with a local building company. He has had a post-aural hearing aid for about 5 years and lip-reads very well.

1   How would you teach a junior nurse to communicate with Mr Bowen?
2   Why might Mr Bowen shout when he is talking?
3   What steps can be taken to ensure that the information gained from Mr Bowen during the admission interview is correct?
4   What should the nursing staff know about caring for a patient with a hearing aid?
5   What are the problems that Mr Bowen faces in the community?
6   What aids and support are available to help Mr Bowen lead an independent life?
7   What might be your response when Mr and Mrs Bowen express concern about their daughter's hearing and ask whether it will develop normally?
8   How would you explain to a junior colleague the difference between conductive and perceptive deafness?

2.3   Answers

1   It is important to find out what the junior nurse already
knows about communicating with the deaf. A discussion
about the subject may be a good idea before showing the
junior nurse how to communicate.

   The junior nurse should then be observed in order to test
that she has learnt.

   The following points should be included in the discussion:
● Methods of communication:
 1 Sign language—hard to learn, qualified interpreter
   needed if this is the only way the individual can communicate
 2 Finger-spelling—quite easy to learn
 3 Written communication
 4 Lip-reading
● As Mr Bowen lip-reads very well, it may be possible to
   use lip-reading only. The points to consider are:
 1 For good lip-reading adequate lighting is essential. Face
   Mr Bowen when talking to him about 5–6 feet away.
 2 Do not move around during the conversation.
 3 Avoid shouting. This distorts the face of the speaker.
 4 Lip movements need to be clear. Speak more slowly than
   normal.
 5 Do not speak with your hand in front of your mouth.
 6 Do not change the subject suddenly.
 7 Be patient.
 8 Avoid the use of jargon; write down medical terms.
 9 Use gestures.
10 Remember Mr Bowen will not be able to do anything
   else when lip-reading, so do not interrupt activities, e.g.
   eating, reading, etc.
11 Attract Mr Bowen's attention before you start talking to
   him.
12 Check that his hearing aid is working.

2   Under normal circumstances we regulate the loudness of
our voices by the way in which we ourselves hear them.
We hear our own voices partly by bone conduction and
partly by air conduction. Mr Bowen has sensori-neural deafness in which the sound of his own voice, and everything
else, is not well conducted by bone. He will probably feel
that he is not talking loud enough and will therefore shout.

3   ● Mr Bowen may be able to fill in some aspects of the form
      himself. This would ensure that the information is correct.

- Show Mr Bowen what you have written in order to confirm the information.
- Involve Mrs Bowen in the interview.

4   It is important to know that hearing aids only amplify sound; they do not select or interpret sound. This means that all background noise is amplified. It is important not to shout.

A hearing aid is most effective when the speaker is not more than 7 feet away from the microphone; beyond this distance the sound fades.

Mr Bowen's aid is one that fits behind the ear. The ear mould needs cleaning weekly in warm soapy water. The hearing aid itself must not come into contact with water. Ensure that Mr Bowen has his hearing aid turned on when you talk to him.

5   The following points should be discussed:
- Inability to hear the doorbell or anyone coming in if the door has been left open
- When walking, inability to hear approaching traffic and footsteps in the dark
- Inability to hear fire alarms, sirens and people shouting about some danger
- Inability to hear radio warnings of, for example, bad weather conditions
- Likelihood of missing day-to-day information, e.g. train cancellations or alterations of platform number
- Difficulty in lip-reading in pubs and restaurants due to subdued lighting and constant movement
- Difficulty in shops or other public places when asking for help or directions and when returning faulty items
- Isolation in social gatherings
- Reception of background noise through the hearing aid in public places
- Difficulty in keeping speech intelligible

6   • The Royal National Institute for the Deaf
- Various aids available from the Royal National Institute for the Deaf, e.g. flashing light alarm clock, visual indicator/baby alarm, fire alarm, flashing light doorbell system
- Sub-titles on television, programmes especially for the deaf and the hard of hearing, play synopsis service
- The British Association of the Hard of Hearing, the British Deaf Association
- Specialized libraries
- Hard-of-hearing clubs

- Induction loop-systems in cinemas, etc., to help people with hearing aids

7   Firstly reassure Mr and Mrs Bowen that this type of deafness is not hereditary and therefore that their daughter's hearing should develop normally. The following tests will be carried out to ensure that her hearing is normal:

(a) First a hearing test is performed at the age of 6–8 months and is normally carried out by the health visitor. She must be able to control her head movements as the test involves turning towards the sound of familiar noises, e.g. rattles.

(b) After this test, yearly hearing tests should be carried out in the community clinic.

(c) Audiometry is carried out as soon after school entry as possible. These tests are performed on all children.

8

Conductive deafness	Perceptive (sensori-neural) deafness
The sound waves fail to reach the inner ear due to a defect in the external ear, middle ear or oval window. In many cases surgery will improve hearing.	This is a disorder of the inner ear, the auditory nerve impulse pathway, or the auditory centre in the brain. Sound waves are therefore not transmitted to the brain.

2.4   Mark Thompson—a young boy with otitis media

Mark Thompson is 10 years old. Over the past 6 months Mark has had several attacks of acute otitis media with throat infections. On each of these occasions his doctor has prescribed antibiotics.

1   What advice could Mr and Mrs Thompson have been given in order to look after Mark at home during these episodes?
2   List the possible complications of otitis media and explain briefly why they can occur.
3   How would the above complications be recognized?

Shortly after the last attack Mark's teacher asks to see his parents. She suggests that he should have his hearing tested as he is inattentive in class and seems to be falling behind with his work. Mark is seen by an ear, nose and throat specialist who diagnoses secretory otitis media ('glue ear'). Audiometry reveals conductive deafness.

4   With reference to normal and altered physiology explain why Mark has developed conductive deafness.

Mark is admitted to the ward as a day case for bilateral myringotomies and insertion of Grommet tubes.

5   What will be the advantages of performing Mark's operation on a day care basis?
6   How could Mark be prepared for surgery following arrival in the ward?
7   What would you tell a junior nurse about the purpose of the operation?

Mark recovers well following surgery and is ready to go home later in the day.

8 What advice and instructions should Mr and Mrs Thompson be given so that they can continue to care for Mark at home?
9 What response should the nurse make when Mrs Thompson rings up 3 weeks later to say that one of the Grommet tubes has fallen out?

2.4   Answers

1
- It is important that Mark takes the whole course of antibiotics, even if he feels well.
- He may be prescribed nasal drops or a decongestant to aid drainage via the Eustachian tube.
- He may also be prescribed eardrops for the relief of pain. They should be instructed how to instil the drops (with the outer ear pulled up and back).
- Mr and Mrs Thompson should always wash their hands before and after contact with the ear, as should Mark.
- When resting, Mark should lie with the affected ear downwards to promote drainage.
- Mild analgesia, e.g. paracetamol, may be given if he is restless or in pain.
- A covered hot-water bottle (the water should be no warmer than 38.9°C) may be placed over the ear to ease discomfort.
- If Mark has a fever he should be kept cool and given extra fluids. Paracetamol will also help to bring down his temperature.
- Mark must stay away from school until he has been seen again by the doctor.

2

- **Acute Mastoiditis** The mastoid processes are full of air cells which communicate with the middle ear. Infection can spread back to them.
- **Chronic otitis media** This can develop if the eardrum perforates causing necrosis of the ossicles and cavity walls.
- **Meningitis** This can occur from spread of infection through the thin roof of the middle ear.
- **Facial paralysis** Chronic infection may affect the facial nerve which lies close to the middle ear.
- **Labyrinthitis** This is the spread of infection to the inner ear.

3
- By pain behind the ear, increasing irritability, pyrexia, swelling, redness, and tenderness over the mastoid area.
- Chronic otitis media is not usually picked up until examination by doctor. Increasing deafness may be an indication.

- Sudden onset of high temperature, headache, lethargy and neck stiffness
- Partial or total loss of the functions of the facial muscles or loss of sensation in the face
- Vertigo—feelings of dizziness, nausea and faintness

4   The hearing part of the ear has two sections:

(a) **Perceiving apparatus** This analyses and interrupts sounds and consists of neuro-epithelial structures.

(b) **Conducting apparatus** This carries sound waves to the

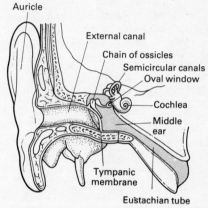

Fig. 4   Cross-section of the middle ear.

perceiving apparatus. It consists of the auricle and the external canal, the tympanic membrane and chain of ossicles, the middle ear cleft, and the perilymph and endolymph of the inner ear. Sound waves are transmitted by vibration of the ossicles and the oval window. For vibration to occur the air pressure must be the same on either side of the tympanic membrane. This is brought into effect by air entering the Eustachian tube from the nasopharynx. Infection in the middle ear causes inflammation and the formation of pus. The Eustachian tube becomes blocked and air is unable to reach the middle ear. The transmission of sound waves is interrupted causing conductive deafness.

5   • It reduces the amount of time spent away from the security of home.
- It enables one or other parent to stay with Mark all day.
- It saves any difficulty parents may have with other children.

- It makes possible economic savings for parents.
- It is more economically viable for the hospital.
- It makes the waiting list shorter.

6 Give him an explanation of the anaesthetic and the operation. He should be told that everything will sound louder
after the operation and he should be given the chance to
ask questions.
- Ensure that he has had nothing to eat or drink for 4 hours
pre-operatively.
- Test his urine for glucose (diabetes) and protein (renal
disorders).
- Ensure that he has an identiband with the correct details
written on it.
- Administer pre-medication as prescribed (if ordered).
- Involve his parents in his care and to keep him company.

7 Myringotomy is the surgical incision of the tympanic membrane to relieve pressure and allow drainage. The small
teflon Grommet tube is inserted through the myringotomy
incision. The purpose of the Grommet tube is to:
- Allow for continuous ventilation of the middle ear
- Drain fluid away from the eardrum into the external
auditory canal
- Equalize the air pressure in the middle ear

The tubes will be left in for up to several months.

8 All instructions should be both verbal and written and
should include:
- Advice regarding the introduction of diet.
- When to return to school.
- Advice to rest and sleep for the first few days following
surgery.
- Advice about the sort of discharge to accept as normal.
There might be blood-tinged discharge for 2/3 days. The
ear should be dry in 3/4 days. Instructions should be
given about what to do if the discharge persists or
becomes thick and yellow, i.e. ring their general practitioner.
- Do not try to remove the tubes.
- Do not allow water to get into Mark's ears as this could
cause infection. Swimming may be allowed if his ears are
plugged, but this depends on the surgeon. Care should be
taken with hair-washing.
- Only the outer part of the ear should be cleansed (with
cotton wool and water).

9 Reassure Mrs Thompson that there is nothing to worry about and that Mark will not come to any harm. Reiterate that the tubes are designed to come out by themselves but usually at a later stage than this. She should not attempt to replace it. She can throw the tube away. There is no urgent need to see the doctor but she should make an appointment so that he can assess the need for reinsertion.

3 Care of the Female Patient and her Reproductive System

3.1   Anne Walsh—a young girl undergoing a termination of pregnancy

> Anne Walsh is a 16-year-old schoolgirl who has been admitted for termination of pregnancy. She is a quiet, shy girl who seems unwilling to enter into any conversation. She is 12 weeks pregnant and is to undergo a vacuum aspiration as a day case.

1   As the nurse assisting Anne on admission, how may you overcome her shyness and encourage conversation?
2   Explain the specific information that should be obtained during the admission assessment.
3   What early features of pregnancy may Anne have already noticed?
4   What are the implications to the nursing profession of the 1967 Abortion Act?
5   What criteria have to be fulfilled to enable a legal termination to be performed?
6   Describe Anne's preparation for theatre.
7   Describe the significance of the observations made of Anne in the immediate post-operative period.
8   Post-operatively Anne becomes very tearful. She says that a friend has told her that abortion is murder. She asks you if the baby is fully formed at 12 weeks. How can you answer?
9   Before discharge Anne asks for an explanation of the different methods of contraception available. What information should be given to her?
10   What other advice should be given to Anne when she is ready for home?

3.1 Answers

1. Although Anne is quiet this does not mean that she does not want to talk; she may find it difficult to express herself. Establish some physical and eye contact with Anne. Placing a hand on her shoulder will indicate reassurance and acceptance. It is important that you do not indicate disapproval, even unintentionally, by facial expression or speech. Ensure that the two of you have privacy for your conversation so that Anne will not be inhibited by fear of being overheard. Try to initiate conversation by asking Anne about herself. Use 'open' questions such as 'How do you like school?' in order to encourage Anne to talk. Discuss such non-threatening subjects first rather than starting by asking her about the reasons for admission.

2. The specific information needed on admission is:
   - **the date of Anne's last normal menstrual period** This will provide a check that she is no more than 12 weeks pregnant. (A suction termination is dangerous if the pregnancy is more advanced than this time.) Check also her normal pattern of menstruation. Has she ever missed periods before? If so, why?
   - **regularity of sexual intercourse** To discover whether the pregnancy was the result of casual sex or the result of a long-standing relationship. Anne may need advice about the dangers of casual sex or advice on contraception if she has a regular boyfriend.
   - **any contraception used** It is important to find out 'what went wrong' with any method of contraception used to prevent further unwanted pregnancies.
   - **parental support** Find out if Anne's parents know about the termination and whether they will support her afterwards. If her parents are unaware of the situation find out if she has anyone else to look after her.
   - **Anne's personal feelings** Is the termination the result of careful consideration or does Anne feel pressurized into making this decision? Anne may need further counselling if she is to avoid feelings of guilt and depression post-operatively.

3. - Enlargement and tingling of her breasts and nipples
   - Prominence of the veins over her breast
   - Darkening of the area around her nipples
   - Nausea and/or vomiting on awaking

4. The Abortion Act (1967) states that no person is obliged to

participate in the termination of a pregnancy if they hold a conscientious objection to such a procedure. Because nurses must participate in treatment that may be necessary to save the life of the patient or prevent injury to the patient undergoing the termination, nurses are advised to request not to be allocated to gynaecological wards or theatres if they would rather not be involved with terminations.

5   Anne must have been examined by two independent doctors who both agree that continuation of the pregnancy would result in a greater risk to:
- Anne's life
- Anne's physical or mental health
- any existing child(ren)'s physical or mental health
- the unborn child who would be born with a serious mental and/or physical handicap

6
- **Basic-line observations** Observations should be carried out of temperature, pulse, respirations and blood pressure to enable a comparison of Anne's post-operative condition with her pre-operative condition to be made.
- **Pubic, vaginal and perineal shave** This depends on the surgeon's policy. If it is necessary Anne may prefer to do this herself but it should be checked by the nurse.
- **Bowel action** Ensure that Anne has a regular bowel action. A full bowel may make surgery difficult because of the proximity of the uterus and bowel. Suppositories may be necessary.
- **Vaginal discharge** Check that Anne has no vaginal infection which could lead to post-operative complications.
- **Haemoglobin** There should be an up-to-date record of Anne's haemoglobin level in case of severe blood loss during or after surgery. The need for transfusion can then be accurately assessed.
- **Consent** Check that Anne has signed her consent form. Be able to consolidate the doctor's explanation for her surgery in order to allay anxiety. (Tell Anne that the entrance to her womb or cervix will be gradually stretched so that the products of conception can be extracted.) The cervix will contract gradually back to shape after the operation. This may cause a pain similar to period pain. She will have a sanitary pad in place when she awakes. (The nurse will check this and her pulse at $\frac{1}{2}$–1 hourly intervals to check that she is not bleeding too heavily.)
- **Nil-by-mouth** This should be the procedure for at least 4–6 hours prior to theatre in order to prevent inhalation

of vomit during anaesthesia. Anne may have come into hospital having been told to fast from midnight.

- **Identiband** This is necessary to ensure that the correct patient receives the correct treatment in the theatre. Anne should also be dressed in a theatre gown, any prosthesis removed, and any valuables locked away.
- **Pre-medication** One hour pre-operatively hyoscine 0.3 mg, for example, should be given to dry up secretions and facilitate anaesthesia, and papaveretum 15 mg should be administered to allay anxiety. Anne's bladder should be emptied prior to this so that she can be left to rest.

7

Observation	Significance
Pulse	A weak, fast pulse would indicate reactionary haemorrhage.
Blood loss	A heavy blood loss per vagina of bright, fresh blood would also indicate a reactionary haemorrhage.
Colour	Extreme pallor may be the first sign of asphyxia.
Respirations	Dyspnoea may be the first sign of asphyxia.
Temperature	A subnormal temperature may indicate shock due to blood loss.

8   Explain to Anne that there are two very different views on abortion. Some people, like her friend, believe that abortion is a form of murder. Others deny this because although the baby is fully formed at 12 weeks it is unable to live a separate existence outside the womb and therefore should not be considered as a living thing.

Some people will also argue that the unborn baby has the right to live. Conversely, the life of a child with adopted parents or with a young single parent must be considered.

Anne has made her decision and this decision must be given full support. She can be told that those who disagree with her are not in her individual situation.

9   Anne should be given a comparison of the different methods of contraception and advised to talk over her contraception with her boyfriend so that they choose a method that suits them both. She should be given advisory leaflets about the various methods. She can also be told that her local family planning clinic will give further advice if necessary.

Method	Description	Action	How used
Pill	Synthetic hormones oestrogen and/or progesterone.	Prevents ovulation.	1 pill daily for 21–26 day cycle. Care if vomiting and/or diarrhoea.
Intrauterine device (IUD)	Small plastic device introduced to the uterine cavity.	Thought to irritate uterine lining and prevent implantation.	Inserted by doctor. Check string weekly. Yearly check-up.
Cap	Circular, flexible rubber dome which lies over the cervix + contraceptive jelly.	Blocks entrance to uterus (while the jelly acts as a spermicide).	Inserted into vagina before intercourse. Must not remove until 6 hours later.
Condom	Thin, rubber sheath.	Collects sperm, thus preventing entry to the vagina.	Rolled on over penis.
Rhythm	Calculation of fertile days 6–7 days prior to ovulation.	Avoidance of intercourse on fertile days.	Temperature measured a.m and p.m. Unsafe when temperature rises.
Chemical barriers	Jelly, cream paste pessaries, aerosol foam/film.	Spermicidal.	Inserted into vagina via an applicator.
Withdrawal	Coitus interruptus.	Prevents entry of sperm into the vagina.	Withdrawal of penis before ejaculation.
Billings method	Calculation of fertile days.	Avoidance of intercourse during the fertile period.	Observation of chemical mucus. Becomes stickier and more profuse during fertile period around time of ovulation.

Contraindications	Advantages	Disadvantages
A family history of thrombosis.	Short, light, pain-free periods (99.9% effective).	Breast enlargement, nausea, weight gain, ?? risk of thrombosis.
Pelvic infection, urine abnormality.	Minimum of effect (97% effective).	Menorrhagia, metrorrhagia expulsion, perforation, infection.
Loss of vaginal tone.	Simple to insert (92% effective).	Allergic response, dislodgement, loss of spontaneity. Re-fit if loss or gain of 10 lbs, and after pregnancy.
Allergy.	Easy (85% effective).	Allergic response, loss of spontaneity, care on withdrawal.
Irregular periods, inability to calculate safe periods.	Acceptable to Roman Catholics (76% effective).	Mental/physical strain, infection, etc.
Allergy.	Easy. Increase effectiveness of condom and cap.	Not very reliable. Best used with cap or condom.
	Always available.	Mental stress. Not reliable.
Needs daily self examination and understanding of principles.	No religious objection.	Not easy. Effectiveness not yet fully evaluated.

Reassure her that she does not have to be married to seek such advice.

Find out what she already knows about the different methods. Then talk through each method with her, discussing the advantages and disadvantages of each of them (as stated in the table on pp. 62 and 63).

10   Anne can go back to school the following week. She should expect some vaginal loss for the next 7–10 days. This should be minimal and dark red or brown in colour. Any variation in this should be reported to her general practitioner.

She should also seek advice from her doctor if she suffers any severe abdominal pain and/or fever.

3.2 Mrs England—a young woman who has had a ruptured ectopic pregnancy

Mrs England, aged 25 years, has been admitted to the ward in a collapsed state. She is accompanied by her husband who is very agitated because they were looking forward to the birth of their first baby. Mrs England has been diagnosed as having had a ruptured ectopic pregnancy and is to be prepared for urgent surgery.
Mr England is anxious to ensure that you realize that his wife's blood group is A rhesus-negative.

1 In priority order, which of the following would be your first 10 actions following Mrs England's arrival on the ward? Give reasons for your choice.
- Elevate the foot of the bed.
- Administer prescribed analgesia.
- Reassure Mr England and give him a cup of tea.
- Observe and record half-hourly pulse and blood pressure measurements.
- Find out when Mrs England last ate.
- Test Mrs England's urine.
- Shave Mrs England's abdominal and pubic area.
- Record Mrs England's fluid balance.
- Help the house surgeon to set up intravenous fluids.
- Reassure Mrs England.
- Explain all care and treatment to Mr and Mrs England.
- Take a nursing history from Mrs England.
- Ensure a consent form has been signed.
- Interview Mr England to obtain admission details.
- Remove any prosthesis.
- Give any jewellery to Mr England for safe-keeping.
- Observe and record Mrs England's temperature and respirations.
- Administer prescribed atropine 0.6 mg.
- Place her gently into a bed near the nurses' station.

2 Mr and Mrs England are obviously anxious and upset. How should the nurse reassure them both initially?

3 What immediate information will the nurse require from Mr England before his wife goes to theatre? Why is this information important?

4   Which one of the following makes urgent surgery necessary for Mrs England? The risk of:
    (a) peritonitis?
    (b) severe haemorrhage?
    (c) pelvic inflammatory disease?
    (d) rupture of the uterus?

5   Why is the information that Mrs England has A rhesus-negative blood group significant?

6   With reference to anatomy and physiology describe the term 'ruptured ectopic gestation' to a junior colleague and explain why Mrs England was in a collapsed state on admission.

7   Mr England asks the cause of his wife's condition. How would you reply?

Mrs England returns from theatre following a right salpingectomy. She has a blood transfusion in progress and the surgeon has asked for an hourly measurement of urine output.

---

8   Explain why an accurate record of urine output is important.

9   With reference to anatomy and physiology explain this operation and its significance to Mrs England.

10 What advice should the nurse give Mrs England before her discharge?

3.2 Answers
1

Action	Rationale
1 Place her gently into a bed near the nurses' station.	The patient is very shocked so she needs careful handling and close observation.
2 Administer prescribed analgesia.	This reduces shock and hypotension which can lead to acute renal failure.
3 Reassure Mrs England.	This reduces shock.
4 Observe and record half-hourly pulse and blood pressure measurements.	This monitors the degree of shock.
5 Help the house surgeon to set up intravenous fluids.	Mrs England needs urgent replacement of fluids to reduce shock.
6 Explain all care and treatment to Mr and Mrs England.	This reassures them, reduces Mrs England's shock and pain, and helps her to cooperate.
7 Find out when Mrs England last ate.	Mrs England needs surgery as soon as possible.
8 Observe and record Mrs England's temperature and respirations.	This monitors the degree of shock and collapse and acts as a pre-operative base-line.
9 Record Mrs England's fluid balance.	This monitors fluid replacement and urine output. (Anuria or oliguria could be the onset of acute renal failure.)
10 Interview Mr England to obtain admission details.	Mrs England is too shocked to be interviewed in depth. Crucial history (such as past medical history) can be gleaned from her husband.

The other aspects of care (*except* elevating the bed end) must be done pre-operatively but are not immediate priorities. Elevating the foot of the bed would cause the build-up of blood in the abdominal cavity, and movement of the diaphragm and heart will be embarrassed by this increase in abdominal contents.

2 Explain that this baby is unfortunately lost but that other babies will be possible. This baby was growing in the wrong place which is why the pregnancy came to an end. This is a fairly common occurrence and although urgent surgery is necessary Mrs England will soon recover.

3 • **Length of pregnancy** This gives a rough idea of fetal size.
  • **Past medical history**
  1 For example, diabetes, a chronic respiratory or cardiac condition, steroid therapy that may cause problems during general anaesthesia
  2 Any previous abdominal surgery, especially gynaecological surgery, which may affect the site of incision or the type of surgery.
  • **Personal details**
  1 Name, address and telephone number to contact Mr England
  2 Religion (in case Mrs England's condition deteriorates)
  3 Mrs England's occupation to enable accurate planning of discharge advice
  4 Name and address of GP to inform him of the admission and treatment.

4 (b). In this situation patients can exsanguinate very quickly. The shock and hypotension caused by the blood loss may also lead to acute renal failure.

5 If Mr England's blood is rhesus-positive (as are 85% of the population) the baby will have had rhesus-positive blood also, as this gene is dominant. As the baby's blood intermingles with Mrs England's blood, her blood will develop antibodies against the foreign rhesus factor. This does not affect the first pregnancy but these antibodies will attack and destroy the blood cells of any further babies. To prevent this, Mrs England must be given anti-D immunoglobulin.

6 Using the diagram opposite to refer to the relevant anatomy explain that an ectopic gestation is a pregnancy that occurs elsewhere than in the uterine cavity. The commonest site for such a pregnancy is the fallopian tube, although ovarian and even peritoneal pregnancies may occur.

   The developing ovum begins to grow within the uterine tube which ruptures when it cannot stretch any further. This is then termed a 'ruptured ectopic gestation'. The patient will then collapse because the rupture of the fallopian tube will cause internal haemorrhage into the peritoneum. This will cause a sudden fall in blood pressure. The severe pain caused by irritation of the peritoneum adds to the patient's collapsed state. The patient will be pale and her

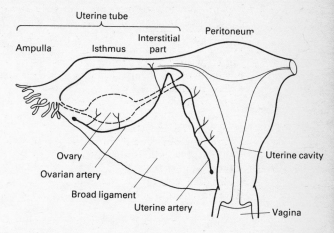

Fig. 5 Cross-section of the female reproductive system.

skin will feel cold and clammy because the blood supply to the periphery is very poor. She may feel faint because of cerebral anoxia. Fear and anxiety may add to her shocked condition. This explanation can be clarified by accompanying the junior nurse to look at Mrs England and comparing her condition with your description.

7   Tubal pregnancies occur about once in every 200–300 pregnancies. Any condition such as salpingitis (inflammation of the uterine tubes) or a congenital deformity of the uterine tube, which narrows the lumen of the tube, may prevent the fertilized egg from passing further into the uterus.

It may be helpful to show Mr England a diagram of the uterus and tubes to facilitate this explanation.

8   An accurate estimation of urine output is important whenever a patient has had a prolonged period of hypotension. In this situation peripheral blood vessels constrict to direct blood to the vital organs. This vasoconstriction causes a marked reduction in renal blood flow. If renal ischaemia is prolonged, acute renal failure may result.

In order to monitor the degree of renal damage, the urinary output is measured hourly. The doctor should be informed if the output falls below 30 ml per hour so that measures can be taken to improve renal perfusion.

9   Show Mrs England the diagram below and explain that a salpingectomy means removal of one of her uterine tubes (in her case the left tube). Because the right ovary and tube have been left intact, her ability to menstruate and become pregnant has not been affected.

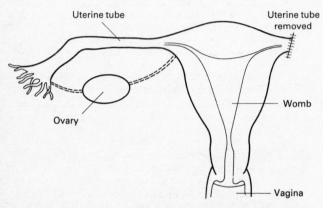

Fig. 6   The female reproductive system following a salpingectomy.

10 • It should be explained to Mrs England that she lost a lot of blood internally and consequently she may feel lethargic for a week or two. She should finish the course of iron tablets which will help her body to replace its red blood cells. These should be taken at meal-times to avoid causing nausea. She will find that her stools are black while she is taking the iron tablets; this is quite normal.
    • She can continue sexual intercourse as soon as she wants to and can try for another baby straight away.
    • She can return to work after a month's convalescence at home.
    • She is likely to experience a feeling of great weariness and sadness, which accompanies any surgery. It will pass as her body returns to normal. She should not be afraid to grieve for her baby.

3.3 Mrs Lomax—a patient with carcinoma of the cervix

Mrs Diana Lomax, aged 40 years, has been admitted to your ward after she was found to have carcinoma of the cervix (stage 1) after a routine cervical smear followed by a cone biopsy.

She is married with a 16-year-old daughter, Claire. She has recently returned to work as a part-time auxilliary nurse in a local old people's home.

It has been decided to treat Mrs Lomax by insertion of caesium followed at a later date by hysterectomy.

1 Describe the specific information the nurse will require when assessing Mrs Lomax on admission.
2 Mrs Lomax says that her mother died of carcinoma of cervix 2 years after extensive surgery. She wants to know if this treatment will be more successful as she is concerned about her family if she does not have long to live. How should the nurse reply?
3 Describe Mrs Lomax's specific preparation for her caesium implant.
4 As the nurse in charge of the ward explain the precautions you should take with regard to:
   (a) the safety of your staff
   (b) Mrs Lomax's visitors
5 Using a problem-solving approach plan Mrs Lomax's specific care while the caesium is in situ.
6 Describe what the nurse-in-charge should do if a source becomes lost.
7 A junior colleague has never seen caesium removed. How should the nurse teach this procedure?
8 Discuss the role of the nurse in relation to educating the public about carcinoma of the cervix.

3.3   Answers

1   The nurse will require information about:
  • **Mrs Lomax's knowledge of her condition and proposed treatment** so that any misconceptions can be explained. Endeavour to observe Mrs Lomax for her emotional response to her diagnosis so that you can support her as necessary.
  • **Mrs Lomax's general physical condition** (nutritional status, weight, other illnesses) to assess how she will respond to treatment.
  • **Mrs Lomax's family relationships**, both supportive and dependent, to ensure that the family can manage without her and can help her on discharge.
  • **her menstrual history** The date of her last normal menstrual period (LNMP) is required as treatment is avoided at the time of menstruation. For menorrhagia, a blood transfusion may be needed before treatment.
  • **her contraceptive history** An intrauterine contraceptive device would need removal prior to treatment. Sudden stoppage of the contraceptive pill would cause withdrawal bleeding.
  • **any vaginal discharge** Any discoloured, offensive discharge may be due to an infection. A swab should be taken so that treatment can commence.

2   The nurse should explain gently to Mrs Lomax that extensive surgery is used as a means of relieving distressing symptoms of invasive carcinoma. Therefore, her mother's cancer had certainly spread outside the cervix before diagnosis. In such cases the average time between the onset of symptoms and death is about 2 years.

   However, in Mrs Lomax's case her cancer has been diagnosed before it has spread outside the cervix. This is why she has no symptoms. In such cases caesium is used to kill the malignant cells, so no further spread is possible before removal of the entire uterus, which doubly ensures that no spread can occur.

   The success rate in such cases is much higher than in her mother's situation.

3   The nurse will need to reinforce the radiotherapist's explanations before Mrs Lomax signs her consent for treatment. It must be explained to Mrs Lomax that she will have to remain on flat bed rest for the 24 hours that the caesium is in situ. Consequently, movement will be limited. Staff and

visitors will only have limited access to her during this time, but she will have a call-bell at hand. She will be sedated over the 48 hours to minimize discomfort.

Before the implant an enema will be given because a bowel action while the caesium is in situ could dislodge the implant. Laxatives are discontinued and a low residue diet commenced. A Foley catheter is inserted to avoid excessive movement when using bedpans.

The day before the implant Mrs Lomax will be able to have a bath and shampoo. Mrs Lomax should be aware that the implant will be inserted in theatre under a general anaesthetic but that it will be removed on the ward.

4 (a) All staff should understand that the intensity of the radiation decreases with the distance from the source. All essential nursing procedures during the treatment should be carried out as quickly as possible, with the nurse keeping as far as is practicable from the source. Each nurse should only remain at the bedside for 2 minutes at a time, and should not spend more than 15 minutes in 24 hours with Mrs Lomax. A record should be kept of each nurse's time spent with the patient. A lead apron should be worn at the bedside.

The nurse-in-charge should ensure that no nurse who is to care for Mrs Lomax is pregnant.

Staff involved in Mrs Lomax's care should be given a film badge to wear. These badges will record each individual's level of radiation.

The statutory radiation warning sign must be placed on the door of Mrs Lomax's side room to remind staff of the hazard and to prevent unauthorized staff from entering the room.

(b) Visitors should be restricted to a 20-minute visiting period each. They should stay mainly at the foot of the bed at a distance of 6 feet. Mr Lomax may wish to be nearer his wife but is limited to 4 feet and may then only stay for 10 minutes.

Claire will not be allowed to visit her mother and pregnant mothers should also be banned from visiting while the caesium is in situ.

5

Problem	Aim	Nursing care	Evaluation
Potential risk of dislodging the implant	To keep Mrs Lomax as still as possible to prevent the implant from dislodging	• Position patient on her back with two or three pillows. Explain that she may only turn on to her side when a nurse is present.	While Mrs Lomax is lying still, implant remains in position.
		• Give a low residue diet (to avoid the necessity for opening her bowels)	Bowels not open
		• Check the position of the implant 2–4 hourly.	
Discomfort of immobility	To ensure that Mrs Lomax is comfortable	• Sponge as necessary	Mrs Lomax says she is comfortable.
		• Change the perineal pad as necessary. Swab the perineal area.	
Potential complications of immobility	To ensure that the skin remains intact To ensure that there is free flow of urine	• Change position 2–4 hourly.	There is no breaking of skin.
		• Give 2–3 litres of fluid daily.	
		• Ensure that the catheter bag is below bladder level.	There is good urine output.
		• Ensure that the catheter tubing is not kinked.	

	To encourage good venous return to prevent clotting	• Encourage deep breathing and leg movement. • Observe any complaints of chest or calf pain.	There are no complaints of calf or chest pains.
Potential adverse reaction to radium	To monitor Mrs Lomax for any adverse effects	• Make 2–4 hourly observations of temperature, pulse and respirations. • Check for vaginal bleeding half-hourly. • Observe for nausea, vomiting, diarrhoea or severe pain.	There are no signs of infection or haemorrhage.
Boredom or depression due to isolation	To reduce the feeling of isolation	• Plan the day's activities and visitors so that Mrs Lomax is not alone for long periods. • Provide reading and the radio as desired. • Give comfort and support when present.	Mrs Lomax does not feel too isolated.

6 • All movement in the ward should be stopped as far as possible. No-one should be allowed to enter or leave the ward.
   • The radiological safety officer or a physicist should be contacted.
   • All dressings, linen and bedpans used by the patient should be checked with a Geiger counter in the sluice. The time of the loss should be noted, the nursing officer informed, and an incident report made.

7 First check the junior colleague's present knowledge of caesium treatment. Ensure that she is aware that the uterine applicator has been inserted through the cervical canal into the uterine cavity. The applicators are secured by a vaginal pack, and the labia are sutured together. The source trains are inserted into the applicators. (A diagram can be shown to her for clarification.)

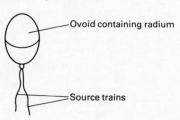

Fig. 7 The caesium implant.

Before the procedure commences, talk it through with the junior nurse. Sedation or analgesia should be given 1 hour before the removal time given in the patient's notes. The procedure should be explained to Mrs Lomax. She will be placed in the dorsal position, and the labial sutures and vaginal pack will be removed. A doctor or physicist will remove the source trains and ovoids and place them in a lead container.

The empty applicators can then be removed by a registered nurse. The time of removal of the implants should be recorded in the patient's notes and nursing records.

The junior nurse should be warned that the vaginal odour may be offensive and she should not indicate this by her facial expression.

The urethral catheter is removed, the vulva swabbed, and a clean perineal pad applied. Continued observation of the patient is necessary as bleeding may occur following removal of the caesium.

The junior nurse may then be asked to help you set up the trolley and assist at the procedure. Allow her time to ask questions afterwards.

8   Nurses should encourage all women who are sexually active to ask for regular (2–3 yearly) cervical smears.

It should be explained that carcinoma of the cervix is one of the most common cancers in women but that treatment is 98–100% successful if it is diagnosed at an early stage.

A cervical smear can diagnose cancer of the cervix at the stage when the cervical cells are abnormal, prior to them becoming malignant.

Such early cancer, if found, is treated by laser minor surgery; removal of a small part of the cervix may be all that is necessary.

The nurse should be aware of the reasons why women do not have regular smears and should try to allay these. Smears are painless and quick. They can be performed at a family planning clinic or by a general practitioner.

Free smear tests can also be done at local well-woman clinics and in mobile units run by the Women's National Cancer Control Campaign. A female nurse or doctor can be requested if embarrassment is a problem.

3.4 Miss Newlands—a young woman expecting her first baby

Jane Newlands, aged 19 years, is expecting her first baby. She is unmarried and lives in a bedsitter in Hackney. She works as a shop assistant in Woolworths. She does not know who is the father of the child and has had no contact with her parents since leaving school at 16 years. She is adamant that she wants to keep the baby.

She has now come for her first ante-natal visit. She is surprised by the number of tests and questions she has been asked. She admits to finding morning sickness a problem.

1 How would you explain to Jane the significance of her first ante-natal visit in relation to:
(a) blood and urine tests?
(b) her physical examination?
(c) the midwife's assessment?

2 What advice should the nurse give Jane with reference to:
(a) diet?
(b) morning sickness?
(c) work?
(d) benefits?

3 Jane is booked for an ultrasound scan. She expresses surprise as she has read that these can be dangerous. How should the nurse respond?

4 As Jane progresses into pregnancy she admits one day to being frightened of the birth. How can the nurse allay her fears?

5 How would you explain to Jane how to recognize the first stages of labour and when to come into hospital.

Jane is delivered of a healthy baby boy at 41 weeks gestation. She had a normal labour and was thrilled to see her new son. She expresses a wish to breast-feed.

6 Explain the significance of the observations you will make of Jane during the puerperal period.

7   What advice should the nurse give Jane about breast-feed-
    ing?
8   How should the nurse teach Jane to care for her baby before
    she is discharged?
9   What advice and support can be given to Jane on discharge?

3.4   Answers

1   (a) Blood will be taken for the haemoglobin level to ensure that Jane is not anaemic during the pregnancy of the baby.

Her blood will be grouped and cross-matched so that blood is ready for transfusion should the need arise. Her resistance to rubella (German measles) will be measured, as exposure to the rubella virus could be risky in early pregnancy if she has not developed a sufficient number of antibodies.

All pregnant women have a routine blood test to discover if they have venereal disease. This could affect the baby unless diagnosed and treated early in pregnancy.

A urine specimen is tested by the nurse to ensure that Jane has no kidney disease or diabetes which could be aggravated by pregnancy.

(b) The doctor or midwife will perform a physical examination to ensure that there are no gross abnormalities. He/she will listen to the heart and lungs to ensure that there are no problems that would be aggravated by pregnancy. Jane's breasts will be examined to ensure there are no lumps and, if she wants to breast-feed, that her nipples are not retracted.

Her blood pressure will be checked as high blood pressure can be a problem during some pregnancies. A record of her weight will help to assess her weight gain throughout the pregnancy. Her abdomen will be palpated to ensure that there are no masses in her abdomen which could hinder the growth of the baby.

A vaginal examination will be performed to ensure that there is no infection present which, if left untreated, could harm the baby at delivery.

(c) The midwife needs to interview Jane to get to know her and so that they can together plan her care during her pregnancy, labour and post-natal care. She will ask about any previous obstetric history as terminations or miscarriages may be relevant to this pregnancy.

The date of the first day of Jane's last normal period helps to determine the expected date of delivery. Contraceptive history is useful to know as the contraceptive pill sometimes makes calculation of this date unreliable.

The midwife will also ask about family and medical history. Some conditions are hereditary and medical problems may need special care during pregnancy. Details of housing, job and finance help the midwife to assess Jane's problems so that she can offer appropriate support.

Her height and shoe size can be helpful in determining her pelvic size and therefore any potential difficulties with a normal delivery.

The midwife will also ask about her smoking and drinking habits, as both nicotine and alcohol can be harmful to her unborn baby. Jane should tell the midwife about any medicine she is taking, as some drugs are not advisable during pregnancy.

2 (a) Jane should not be tempted to eat for two. She will, however, need to eat a well-balanced diet of protein, carbohydrate and fats. She can be given a booklet to give her examples of such foods. An appointment can be made with the dietician if necessary.

She will be given an iron supplement to take once daily. This sometimes causes constipation, which is also a problem anyway for some women during pregnancy. Therefore, Jane should be sure to drink 2–3 litres of fluid (5–6 pints) daily and eat a high fibre diet.

The average expected weight gain during pregnancy is 9 kg (21 lb). Jane will be weighed at each clinic visit so that her weight can be monitored.

(b) Jane should be reassured that morning sickness is a common complaint in the early months of pregnancy but that it usually disappears by 12 weeks. She should be advised to get up slowly. She could take some dry biscuits and a thermos flask of tea or iced water up to bed with her and take these in the morning before getting up. If she does vomit she should try to drink some water afterwards so that she replaces her lost fluid. Deep breathing sometimes helps to control feelings of nausea.

If she continues to find it a problem she should seek advice either from her general practitioner or from the clinic. Medicines are not usually prescribed as they can be dangerous to the baby.

(c) Advice regarding employment will depend on Jane's exact job in Woolworths. She should avoid lifting heavy weights, especially in the first 3 months of her pregnancy. She should also avoid standing still for long periods as this can predispose to varicose veins and piles. Alternate relaxation and contraction of her calf muscles is a useful exercise if she does a lot of standing. In this case, a walk at lunch-time is also beneficial.

She may find she becomes tired in the later months of

pregnancy and may need to reorganize her usual routine to allow for a rest either at lunch-time or when she first gets home.

She is entitled to maternity benefit if she finishes work at week 28 of her pregnancy. She will also leave work at this time if she is going to take maternity leave. She can stay on until the end of her pregnancy but this is not advisable as she will find that she needs more rest in the last 2 months of her pregnancy.

If Jane is not intending to return to work full time she may be eligible for supplementary benefit and help towards housing and heating costs. Jane is also entitled to time off work with pay to attend her ante-natal appointments.

(d)

Benefit	Details
Maternity grant	• A lump sum can be obtained from the Department of Health and Social Security for all pregnant women (who have lived in the country for at least 6 months in the year before the birth). • A claim can be made from week 26 of pregnancy–3 months after delivery.
Maternity allowance*	• A weekly payment is made for 18 weeks (from week 29 of pregnancy to 7 weeks after delivery.) • A claim can be made at week 26 from social security.
Free prescriptions and National Health Service	• These are given throughout pregnancy and up until the baby is 1 year old.
Free dental treatment	• A form should be filled in from the doctor or dentist.
Child benefit	• A monthly cash payment is made until the child has left full-time school. • A claim can be made from social security after registering the baby's birth.
One parent benefit	• An extra payment for single parents is usually paid with the child benefit. • A claim can be made after registering the baby's birth.

* From March 1987, this will be replaced by Statutory Maternity Pay for any woman who has been employed for at least 26 weeks by the 15th week of her pregnancy.

3 An ultrasound scan is a useful, accurate measurement of the size of the baby and can also diagnose gross abnormalities, some of which can be treated. It is quite painless—an instrument like a microphone is passed over the abdomen. A computer converts the sound waves picked up into a picture of the fetus.

American research has shown that multiple ultrasound scans in animals can cause chromosome abnormalities. No research has been done with humans as yet so there is no proof that there is any risk for human fetuses. Ask Jane what she has read. Jane is only booked for one routine scan, so she need have no fears for the safety of her baby. However, if she is still doubtful she has the right to refuse the investigation.

4 Ask her exactly what she is frightened of. If it is pain you can discuss the various methods of pain relief (relaxation, gas and air, pethidine, epidural); she might use a combination of some of these methods. She may be frightened of being alone. Reassure her that a nurse will remain with her throughout the labour.

She may worry that the birth will be very hospitalized and that her wishes will not be considered. Explain that, as far as possible, the midwives will allow her to control the situation. A visit to the ward and delivery room may help to reassure her and allow her to see the equipment and its uses.

Relaxation classes can be offered as another means of helping to allay her fears.

5 The first stage of labour is from the beginning of contractions to full dilatation of the cervix. It may start in one of three ways:

1 the onset of *regular* contractions (rather similar to period pains)
2 breaking of the waters—a sudden release of the amniotic fluid
3 a 'show' of mucus—a release of the plug at the entry of the cervix.

Jane should ring the hospital when any *one* of these events occurs and they will arrange for an ambulance to bring her into the ward.

6

Observation	Significance
Temperature and pulse	A pyrexia and tachycardia may mean that Jane has a puerperal infection.
Lochia	Any greenish-yellow discharge will indicate an infection.
Breasts	Check that Jane's breasts are not engorged with milk. Once she starts breast-feeding check for cracks and soreness, which may mean she should rest that breast for a while.
Size of uterus	The uterus should involute about 1.6 cm per day until the twelfth puerperal day.
Urinary output	Difficulty in micturition can occur due to a fall in the progesterone level and irritation of the pelvic floor muscles.

7   It will take 36–48 hours after delivery for Jane's milk to come down. Until then her breasts will secrete colostrum—a watery fluid which contains valuable antibodies for the baby.

Jane should put her baby to the breast for 2 minutes on each side at first. The midwife will help her to encourage the baby to suck the nipples. Her nipples should be clean and dry before commencing and Jane should be comfortable in a lying or sitting position.

Each day Jane can gradually increase the time her baby is at the breast until he is feeding for about 10 minutes from each breast. However, the length of time is not crucial; baby will decide how long he wants to feed. To stop the baby sucking Jane can gently slide her finger into the baby's mouth.

It is probably better to feed the baby when he wants to be fed, and gradually he will settle into a routine. As long as the baby is gaining weight, is contented and has a wet nappy at changing time, Jane need not worry that he is not getting enough milk.

Jane can be shown how to express milk from her breasts if they become very swollen and painful. This can be kept in the fridge to be given in a bottle later that day if she wants to go out.

A firm, adjustable bra is advisable during breast-feeding

to support the breasts. Breast pads can be tucked into the cups to soak up leaking milk.

Jane may find that she experiences abdominal pains, rather like period pains, while breast-feeding. This is normal and occurs because breast-feeding helps the womb to contract back to its normal size.

8   Jane will need to know how to feed, dress and bathe her baby. She should be shown how to make up a bottle feed and sterilize the equipment in case she should need to use this once she returns home. The nurse should demonstrate this procedure, giving reasons for all the steps. A leaflet can be given to Jane as reinforcement of the instructions.

At first Jane can be shown how to 'top and tail' her baby. The nurse can then watch Jane do this until Jane seems competent and safe. A demonstration of a baby bath can also be given by the nurse who can then watch Jane do this on her own. She should be shown how to keep the umbilical stump clean and dry and how to place the nappy below the stump.

During these demonstrations the nurse can also give general advice on baby care. For instance, up until the age of 3 months babies can become cold very easily, so they should not be exposed unnecessarily. Their room should be kept at an even temperature (about 18°C or 65°F).

When she takes the baby out he should be dressed warmly. A woolly hat, mittens, bootees and a coat are needed, even in the pram with the hood up.

9   • **General health** At first Jane should be advised to relax and not to try too hard. She will find it difficult to adjust to a new routine with the baby, so household chores should be minimized.

   She should try to rest during the day when the baby is asleep so that she does not become overtired.

   • **Exercise** Jane should not forget her post-natal exercises, which will help her to regain her figure and tighten up her pelvic muscles.

   • **Diet** Jane should not try to slim while she is breast-feeding as this uses up a lot of energy. She should continue the well-balanced diet she was advised to eat during pregnancy. She should ensure that she drinks at least 4 pints of fluid a day.

   • **Sex** There is no physical reason why Jane cannot resume sexual intercourse as soon as she wants. She should seek advice about contraception 6 weeks after the birth.

   • **Emotions** Jane should be advised that it is not unusual to feel low-spirited after having a baby. Usually such feelings only last for a day or two, but sometimes they go on for longer. If Jane finds such feelings become overwhelming she should talk to a friend or her health visitor/midwife.

- **Post-natal check-up** Jane should visit her general practitioner about 4–6 weeks after the baby's birth for a check-up. He will check her weight, urine and blood pressure, and perform a vaginal examination to see if her womb and its surrounding muscles are returning to normal.
- **Registration** Jane must register her baby's birth within 6 weeks from the birth date. The registrar will give her a birth certificate which she will need to claim child benefits.
- **Vaginal loss** Jane should expect to continue to have a brownish discharge for some weeks, although this will gradually become less. She should use sanitary towels because tampons may cause infection.

While she is breast-feeding she may not have another period until she stops feeding.

3.5 Mrs Leonard—a patient having vaginal surgery

Mrs Leonard is a 40-year-old housewife who has been admitted to the ward for an anterior and posterior colporrhaphy (Manchester repair) in 2 days time.

She lives with her husband, Ronald, who is a computer programmer. Their family are now grown up and have left home. Susan, aged 18 years, is at University, Stephen, aged 19 years, is in the Navy, and Sylvia, aged 21 years, is married and in the seventh month of her first pregnancy.

Over the last 10 months Mrs Leonard found her prolapse more and more troublesome. When it began to interfere with her usual activities she went to her general practitioner for advice.

1   During her admission interview Mrs Leonard confides that she dreads another vaginal examination. How can you reassure her?

2   With reference to anatomy and physiology how would you explain to Mrs Leonard how the proposed surgery will help to relieve her symptoms?

3   Using a problem-solving approach plan Mrs Leonard's care in the 48 hours prior to surgery.

Mrs Leonard returns from theatre following a vaginal repair. She has a urethral catheter in situ for free drainage.

4   List the specific actual and potential problems of this type of surgery. Why are these problems specific to vaginal surgery?

5   Explain how Mrs Leonard can be helped to successfully regain control of micturition.

6   Describe how Mrs Leonard's pain might be relieved.

7   Explain how Mrs Leonard can be helped to regain her normal bowel habits.

8   During a visit Mrs Leonard's daughter, Sylvia, asks you what she should do to prevent a prolapse in later years. What advice can she be given?

9   Describe the advice Mrs Leonard should be given on discharge.

3.5   Answers

1   First, the nurse must find out what is specifically frightening or embarrassing Mrs Leonard. She can then find ways of lessening the fear or embarrassment. For example, if Mrs Leonard is frightened of the discomfort of the examination, the nurse can explain the procedure and show her some deep breathing and relaxation exercises.

   If embarrassment is a problem the nurse should explain that she will be present throughout the examination and will ensure that her modesty is protected and that she is not unnecessarily exposed.

   It may also help to reassure Mrs Leonard if she knows why the examination is necessary—for the surgeon to assess the degree of prolapse and to ensure that there is no vaginal infection present which may have an adverse effect on post-operative healing.

2   Show Mrs Leonard a diagram (see Fig. 8) to illustrate the

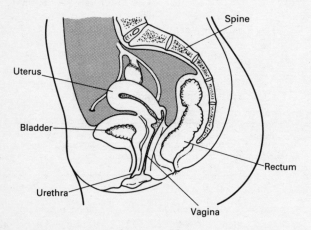

Fig. 8   Cross-section of the female pubic region.

normal anatomy of the pubic area. Due to weakness of the muscles of the floor of the pelvis, probably caused from having her three children, her uterus has slipped downwards. She may be able to feel this prolapse as a lump in her vagina, especially when straining.

   Anteriorly, the prolapsed uterus alters the position of the bladder and this causes her to leak urine when laughing or coughing. Posteriorly, pressure on the rectum may lead to constipation. Sexual intercourse may be painful due to the altered position of the pelvic organs.

An anterior colporrhaphy means that the vaginal wall is excised anteriorly and that the supporting tissue is sutured into the correct position. This will relieve her bladder symptoms. A posterior colporrhaphy repairs the posterior vaginal wall to relieve the rectal symptoms. These repairs will allow the uterus to return to its correct position, relieving sexual problems, and she will no longer be able to feel the prolapse.

3

Problem	Aim	Nursing care	Evaluation
Patient unaware of what surgery entails	To allow Mrs Leonard to make an informed consent	• Explain what an anterior and posterior colporrhaphy entails (as above).	Mrs Leonard was able to understand her proposed operation and was able to sign her consent form confidently.
Potential post-operative problems	To help to prevent:		
	asphyxia due to inhalation of vomit or oral secretions	• Ensure nil-by-mouth for 4–6 hours pre-operatively. • Give prescribed pre-medication 1 hour pre-operatively.	Nothing taken orally for 4–6 hours before surgery. Pre-medication given.
	primary haemorrhage due to vascular endometrium	• Ensure that the menstrual period is not due.	Period not due.

clotting problems	• Teach breathing and leg exercises. Advise no smoking.	Able to carry out breathing and exercise. Not smoking.
	• Check that the contraceptive pill, if used, has been stopped.	Pill stopped 1 month ago.
delayed healing due to infection of operation site	• Give prescribed antibiotics with pre-medication.	Antibiotics given with pre-medication.
	• Shave Mrs Leonard in the pubic, vaginal and perineal area.	Shaved cleanly.
	• Bath before operation. Give a clean gown and bedclothes.	Mrs Leonard had a bath.
	• Give prescribed aperient or suppositories the night before surgery.	Bowels open pre-operatively.
	• Take mid-stream specimen of urine and high vaginal swab.	Specimens taken.
	• Observe urine and any vaginal discharge for signs of infection.	No obvious signs of infection.

Potential discharge problems	To ensure that any difficulties at home are solved before discharge	• Check Mrs Leonard's home situation. Plan convalescence if help is not available.	Mrs Leonard can stay with her daughter after discharge.
Possible other medical problems	To detect any other medical problems	• Carry out a urinalysis. • Check temperature pulse, respirations and blood pressure.	No abnormalities found on urine testing. Vital signs are within the normal limits.
Potential dangers in theatre	To ensure that Mrs Leonard and her belongings are safe while she is in theatre	• Remove any prosthesis. • Dress in operation hat and gown. • Lock away any valuables. • Check that the identiband is correct.	Pre-operative checklist completed.

4

Problems	Reasons
Actual Pain and discomfort	Area of surgery makes the perineal area sore and uncomfortable.
Potential Reactionary haemorrhage	The pelvic area is very vascular.
Retention of urine and urinary infection	The area of surgery is so near the bladder and urethra that these may be damaged during surgery. The patient may find it difficult to urinate at first because of the

	tightened musculature. Retention of urine predisposes to infection as the urine lies stagnant in the bladder.
Clotting disorders (deep vein thrombosis, pulmonary embolus)	Large pelvic vessels are handled in the area of surgery. The lithotomy position used during surgery may interfere with circulation.
Poor wound healing	The vaginal wound is a difficult area to keep clean. It can be contaminated by urine and/or faeces.

5   The Foley catheter should be checked at least hourly to ensure that the urine is flowing satisfactorily. The tubing and Uri-bag should be checked for kinks and the Uri-bag should always be below the level of the bladder.

A urine infection could delay the return of normal micturition when the catheter is removed, so all care should be taken to avoid the entry of infection. The urethral meatus should be cleared twice daily and the catheter bag emptied before it becomes too full. When emptying the bag, the nurse's hands and the receiver should be clean and dry. The urine should be checked for signs of infection (fishy smell, dark colour, presence of pus).

Before the catheter is removed it may be clamped to allow the bladder to fill and regain muscle tone. However, the clamp must be released every 4 hours to prevent over-distension of the bladder which would weaken the repair.

After the catheter is removed (2–4 days post-operatively) the nurse should measure the frequency and amount of Mrs Leonard's micturition. A catheter may be passed after she has urinated to determine whether her bladder has fully emptied. If more than 100 ml of urine is found, the catheter may be left in place for 24–48 hours.

On return from theatre Mrs Leonard should be encouraged to drink 2–3 litres of fluid daily as soon as she is able. It should be explained that this will help to produce a good flow of urine, minimizing the risk of urinary infection. The patient can also be taught perineal exercises by the physiotherapist and nurse to help her regain bladder control.

6   On return from theatre Mrs Leonard should be positioned on her side. When she has fully recovered from the anaesthetic she can be sat up on one side to encourage full chest expansion and to prevent a chest infection. Later she can sit up on an air-cushion.

Intramuscular Omnopon 10–20 mg may be given in the immediate post-operative period and the night following surgery tablets of Temgesic may be effective after this period. If the area is very sore a heat pad or ice-pack may be useful provided that the weight of these appliances is not on the patient.

Once she is mobile the use of a bidet (or vulval wash-downs) may be soothing as well as preventing cross-infection from urine or the bowel. Saline baths may also be comforting.

The use of methods of relieving pain should always be evaluated as pain is so subjective. Mrs Leonard should be asked if pain relief is effective. Her facial appearance and ability to move should also be observed. If pain is still troublesome her care should be altered.

7   Post-operatively there is a danger that faeces will contaminate the wound and that straining will weaken the repair. Therefore, initially Mrs Leonard's diet may be low in residue. (The rectum will have been cleared preoperatively.) Thereafter Mrs Leonard will be advised to continue to drink 2–3 litres daily and to eat plenty of fibre (bran, fresh fruit and vegetables, wholemeal bread) to prevent constipation.

8   Sylvia can be reassured that improved obstetric care before, after and during delivery has now reduced the incidence of prolapse due to childbirth. Prolonged labour and unrepaired tears are no longer likely to happen. However, she can further reduce the likelihood of a prolapse by practising the exercises that she will be taught after delivery of her baby. These have the effect of tightening all the muscles of the pelvic floor.

9   Mrs Leonard should be advised to return to the outpatient department in 6 weeks time for a check-up. Until this time she should avoid lifting anything heavier than a full kettle, standing for longer than half an hour at a time, and prolonged or strenuous exercise. She should avoid constipation. It is safe to resume intercourse about 5 weeks after surgery, but the doctor may ask her to wait until he has seen her in the outpatient department. It may be a little sore initially, so she should ask her husband to be gentle at first.

If Mrs Leonard is still menstruating she should be advised that it is still possible for her to become pregnant and that she will need to use some means of contraception (except the cap at first).

3.6 Mrs Garrod—a young woman with salpingitis

Mrs Lesley Garrod, aged 25 years, is admitted with acute generalized abdominal pain. She is also pyrexial (a temperature of 38.8°C) and feels generally unwell. She has a purulent vaginal discharge. A diagnosis of acute salpingitis is made.

Lesley has been married for 4 years, but has no children. Her husband is in the Navy and has just returned to his ship.

1 Explain the information required from Mrs Garrod during her nursing assessment.
2 Plan Mrs Garrod's care for the first 24 hours in hospital.
3 With reference to anatomy and physiology how would you explain this condition and its possible long-term effects to a junior colleague?

Urethral and vaginal swabs reveal that Mrs Garrod has gonococcal salpingitis. Ampicillin is prescribed. The consultant explains the diagnosis to Lesley and asks how he can contact her husband.

4 What precautions should be taken to limit the spread of this infection in the ward?
5 Why is it important to contact Mr Garrod?
6 List the potential side-effects of ampicillin. What actions should be taken if these occur?
7 How might you reassure Mrs Garrod, who is very upset by the diagnosis?
8 What advice should be given to Mrs Garrod when she is ready for discharge?

3.6   Answers

1   In order to plan Mrs Garrod's care the following information
will be needed:
   - Observe her respirations. Is her abdominal pain affecting
   her breathing?
   - How much is she managing to eat and drink? Is nausea
   a problem?
   - Has the act of passing urine or faeces been a problem?
   (Pyrexia and anorexia may lead to constipation. If the
   urinary tract is also affected, micturition may be painful.)
   - Is her pain and discomfort affecting her ability to move
   around, sleep and rest? What position does she find most
   comfortable?
   - Take her temperature. Ask her if she feels hot or chilly
   so that the bedclothes, etc., may be adjusted accordingly.
   - Ask her about her vaginal discharge. How often does she
   need to change her sanitary pad? Does she find the smell
   offensive?
   - Observe her generally. Does she seem very nervous or
   anxious or is she well-composed and able to express
   herself well?
   - Does she have a job? Are there any financial problems
   due to her admission?

2

Problem	Aim	Nursing	Evaluation
Abdominal pain	To reduce her pain to acceptable levels	• Provide intramuscular analgesia as prescribed. • Use a heat pad.	Mrs Garrod says her pain is no longer a problem.
Pyrexia	To reduce her temperature to normal ranges	• Keep the patient at rest. • Encourage 2–3 litres of fluid daily. • Keep the environment cool with a fan or open window (no draughts).	Her temperature has fallen to 37°C.

	To monitor her pyrexia	● Take 4-hourly temperature checks.	
Vaginal discharge	To encourage drainage and prevent ascending infection	● Sit patient in upright position.	
	To ensure Mrs Garrod's comfort	● Change sanitary towels 1–2-hourly and after bedpan use.	The patient says that discharge is no longer a discomfort.
		● Offer vulval washes when changing towels.	
		● Get Mrs Garrod up for a daily bath.	
		● Use a deodorant as desired.	
Potential complications of immobility	To prevent: thrombosis and embolus	● Encourage breathing and leg exercises.	There are no complaints of chest or calf pains.
	urine retention and constipation	● Encourage fluids (2–3 litres daily).	The urine output is good and the bowels open normally.
	pressure sores	● Encourage movement in bed.	The pressure area is intact.

3 Salpingitis is the term for inflammation of the uterine tubes. The infection is almost always bilateral. The infection may ascend from the uterine cavity, spread via the bloodstream, or result directly from a pelvic peritonitis.

The infection organism causes inflammatory changes within the tubes. The mucosal linings thicken as a result. Local oedema occurs as exudate leaks from capillaries in the area. The exudate usually escapes via the vagina.

The inflammatory response causes Mrs Garrod's pyrexia.

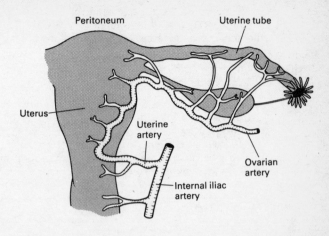

Fig. 9 Cross-section of the female reproductive system (simplified).

The oedema presses on nerve fibres and gives rise to acute abdominal pain.

Salpingitis may be caused by a post-abortal infection or gonorrhoea, or it may be due to a peritoneal infection such as appendicitis or tuberculosis.

Long-term effects If exudate cannot escape, a tubal abscess may form which will need a laparotomy to excise.

If acute salpingitis does not completely resolve, a chronic condition may result with a low-grade infection resulting.

Fibrosis of the tubes may occur as a result of the healing of the inflammatory reaction. This may cause problems of infertility.

4   Gonorrhoea is only spread by sexual intercourse, so isolation precautions are not necessary to prevent the spread of Mrs Garrod's infection on the ward. The unnecessary use of gloves and gowns may cause Mrs Garrod to feel rejected and dirty.

However, because the organism can be spread via the bloodstream it is advisable for the nurse to wear gloves when changing Mrs Garrod's sanitary pad or cleaning her vulval area. The pad should be discarded wrapped in a bag and sent for incineration. Because the gonococcus can also cause blindness, both the patient and the nurse should be especially careful to wash their hands after coming into contact with the vaginal discharge.

Soiled linen should be treated as infected linen although the gonococcus dies rapidly when dry, so spread via linen is very unlikely.

Mrs Garrod should be bathed last if using a general bath, and the bath cleaned and dried after use.

5   The main reason for contacting Mr Garrod is to treat him, as he will almost certainly also have gonorrhoea. He will also need to be asked if he is likely to either have caught the infection from a source other than his wife, or if he has transmitted it further. Any such contacts will need to be treated. He must be warned not to have sexual intercourse until his treatment is complete.

6

Potential side-effect	Action
Anaphylactic shock	Call the cardiac arrest team.
Rash	Inform the doctor. Withhold the next dose until the patient has been examined as it may indicate an allergy.
Vomiting and diarrhoea	Check when ampicillin is given. This effect can be minimized if the drug is given before meals. Inform the doctor if the symptoms become intractable as the drug will no longer be absorbed or effective.

7   The nurse should ensure that she is non-judgemental and shows acceptance of Mrs Garrod to enable the patient to confide in her.

It may be that Mrs Garrod is upset either because she has had sex with another person or because her husband is the cause of her condition. The nurse cannot correct either situation but she can help by listening and giving Mrs Garrod an opportunity to express her feelings. This will also enable the nurse to discover the reason for Mrs Garrod's distress.

Privacy during this conversation is essential so that Mrs Garrod is not afraid to reveal confidential information.

8   Mrs Garrod should be told that it is important that she finishes her course of antibiotics if treatment is to be successful. She should avoid sexual intercourse until treatment is complete.

She should avoid the use of tampons until her discharge has settled as tampons are more likely to encourage ascending infection.

She should not be afraid or embarrassed to seek help should she suspect a recurrence of her symptoms.

4 Care of the Patient with Problems of the Renal and Urinary Systems

4.1 Mr Whittacker—an adult having a urinary diversion

Mr Alan Whittacker, aged 56 years, was admitted to the ward 3 days ago for investigation of painless haematuria. A diagnosis of carcinoma of the bladder has been made and a cystectomy and ileal diversion have been scheduled for 5 days time.

Mr Whittacker is married with two children, both of whom live away from home. He enjoys an active life, playing golf regularly and swimming at least twice a week. Mrs Whittacker works full time.

1 How can Mr Whittacker be helped to begin to accept the forthcoming surgery and the effects it may have on his future lifestyle?
2 Identify the specific pre-operative preparations Mr Whittacker will require in relation to:
  (a) selection of the stoma site
  (b) bowel preparation

Mr Whittacker returns from theatre with an intravenous infusion in progress. He is to have one unit of whole blood followed by dextrose saline. A nasogastric tube is in situ and a transparent, disposable urinary stoma bag has been applied.

3 Identify, giving reasons, the nurse's responsibilities before, during and after the administration of the unit of whole blood.

Two hours following surgery you note that Mr Whittacker's stoma has become a dusky red-blue colour.

4 What is the significance of this observation and what actions should be taken?

Mr Whittacker's wife visits him post-operatively and is keen to participate in his care.

5   What explanation would you give when she asks why he is allowed nothing to eat or drink?
6   Draw up a teaching plan that will enable Mr Whittacker to become able to care for his stoma on discharge.

On the tenth day post-operatively the skin sutures are removed, followed on the fourteenth day by removal of the tension sutures. Mr Whittacker is now eating and drinking well and should shortly be ready for discharge.

7   What advice should Mr Whittacker be given regarding:
    (a) where to obtain appliances?
    (b) how to dispose of appliances?
    (c) the continuation of his hobbies?
8   Identify three possible problems that might occur following discharge and briefly describe the actions Mr Whittacker should take.
9   Where might Mr Whittacker find help and support within the community once he has been discharged from hospital?

4.1   Answers

1   • Give him an explanation of the normal anatomy and function of the bladder.
   • Give him an explanation of the necessity for diverting the urine and how this is done.
   • He must be told that he will in fact be impotent following surgery as the nerves that cause an erection are the same ones that supply the bladder to control the passage of urine. These nerves will have been cut during removal of the bladder. This will be extremely distressing to him and he must be given time to digest this information. His wife will need to be included in discussions. The doctors should explain about the possibility of penile implants following initial surgery. All staff must be sensitive to the impact that impending impotence will have on Mr and Mrs Whittacker.
   • Arrange for the stoma nurse to visit and discuss future management and give reassurance regarding golf and swimming.
   • It may be beneficial for him to talk to somebody who has already undergone the operation. This must be based on individual needs.
   • Be available to listen to his fears and encourage him to talk. Involve his wife in all discussions should he wish to do so.

2   (a) The doctor or stoma nurse will select the stoma site. The site will need to be checked while Mr Whittacker is lying down, sitting and standing. The skin must be free of scars, wrinkles, depressions and skin folds in order for the appliance to be applied adequately. The stoma is not sited on the waistline as it would expose the stoma to excessive pressure from clothing. Several types of skin adhesives will be applied to the abdomen to determine allergies. Mr Whittacker may be encouraged to wear the intended appliance filled with water to simulate urine in order to ensure that the site chosen is a correct one. When the site has been decided upon it will be marked with an indelible marker.
   (b) Mr Whittacker will be given a low residue diet and may be given fluids only for 24 hours before the operation. Enemas will be given as directed for mechanical cleansing of the lower bowel. Antimicrobial agents, e.g. neomycin, may be ordered to reduce pathogenic bacterial flora.

3   • Check the bag of blood with another nurse. You should

check the:
1 patient's identity
2 blood group
3 number of the unit of blood
4 expiry date
with the patient's notes, blood match form and the patient. The purpose of this is to ensure that Mr Whittacker is given compatible blood. Contents of the bag should be checked for particles.

- If dextrose saline is in progress set up a new giving set to administer the blood, as dextrose will cause coagulation of the blood.
- Take Mr Whittacker's blood pressure, pulse and temperature prior to the commencement of the blood to serve as a base-line.
- During the blood transfusion monitor Mr Whittacker's temperature, pulse and blood pressure hourly or as directed to detect any of the following complications:
1 haemolytic reaction—a sudden fall in blood pressure during the first hour of administration
2 febrile reaction—a rise in the temperature
3 allergic reaction—a rise in the temperature and pulse rate
4 circulatory overload—a rise in the pulse rate and respirations
5 infection—a rise in the temperature
- Monitor intake and output.
- On completion of the unit of blood, flush through with normal saline and then continue with the dextrose saline.
- Return the empty blood pack to pharmacy.

4 This indicates that the blood supply to the stoma has become interrupted. This is caused by constriction of the vessels in the root of the mesentery supplying the conduit. This observation must be reported to the doctor immediately as a return to theatre may be necessary.

5 Explain to Mrs Whittacker that under normal circumstances food and fluid is digested and absorbed along the gut or intestines. At the same time it is moved along the gut by a series of rhythmic contractions which squeeze the contents from one portion of the gut to the next.

During the type of surgery that her husband has undergone, the bowel has had to be handled and cut. Excessive handling of the bowel usually causes the rhythmic contractions to cease. Food substances are therefore not moved on through the bowel. Thus, it is necessary to stop Mr

Whittacker's oral intake until the bowel begins to move again. In the meantime fluid will be given by the intravenous infusion.

Reassure Mrs Whittacker that this is a normal occurrence following this type of surgery and that he will be able to begin eating again in about 2–3 days time. Involve her in mouth care.

6 The teaching will have begun pre-operatively and should be built on in conjunction with the stoma nurse. Teaching sessions should be short and held a couple of times a day. The nurse changing Mr Whittacker's appliance should be well versed with the procedure in order to instil confidence. The following plan could be used to enable him to care for his stoma on discharge:

- In the initial post-operative period Mr Whittacker may not be ready to begin learning. During this period, the nurse will change and empty appliances. Encourage him to talk and verbalize his fears.
- Assess his reactions and gradually encourage him to look at the stoma and watch the nurse care for it.
- As he begins to show more interest give him the opportunity to participate.
- Utilize visual aids, e.g. booklets, diagrams.
- Build on his knowledge daily. This may need repetition as anxiety may preclude assimilation.
- Assess how much he is learning by asking questions.
- He must be able to assume self-care before he leaves hospital and must therefore be given the opportunity to practise.
- Encourage the involvement of Mrs Whittacker in the teaching programme.

7 (a) Mr Whittacker must be given the names and serial numbers of the appliances he will be using. His general practitioner will give him a prescription which he can take to a local chemist or to an appliance supplier who will obtain the relevant equipment. He should fill in an exemption form so as not to have to pay prescription charges.

(b) None of his appliances should be flushed down the toilet as they will block the system. They may be disposed of by:

1 burning them on an open fire
2 cutting them into small pieces and then flushing
3 rinsing them clean, wrapping them tightly in a newspaper or plastic bag, and placing them in a dustbin

4 a collection being made by the Department of Environ-
mental Health on request.

(c) There is absolutely no reason for him to give up either
of his hobbies. He may resume both when he is fit.

Small pouches are available to use when swimming. The
pouching may be strengthened by the addition of water-
proof tape.

8

Problem	Action
Infection— indicated by cloudy, offensive urine	Mr Whittacker should increase his fluid intake. If he has a temperature, pain or chills he should contact his doctor.
Blood in the urine	The stoma may bleed very easily; this is quite normal and should stop. However, if it persists it should not be ignored. He should consult his doctor.

Skin irritation which may be due to:
 • allergy
 • the repeated removal of appliances
 • the gasket of the appliance being too big
 • leakage
 • inflammation of the hair follicles
	Refrain from using the product and contact the stoma nurse.
	 Ideally, appliances should be left in position for 3–7 days.
	   Only one-eighth of an inch of clearance between the stoma and the gasket is required. It must not be too tight. Advice should be sought from the stoma nurse.
	   Regular shaving of hairs should help.

9   • general practitioner
     • stoma nurse
     • Urinary Conduit Association
     • sexual counselling clinics
     • social worker

4.2   Mr Clements—a patient having a nephrectomy

Mr John Clements, aged 45 years, has been admitted to the ward for a right nephrectomy for staghorn calculus.

Mr Clements is married with two young children. He is self-employed and his wife has an evening part-time job. They live in a three-bedroomed semi-detached house 20 miles away from the hospital. Mrs Clements does not drive.

On admission, Mr and Mrs Clements voice their fears about how the loss of a kidney will affect his life.

1   What response would you make to them in order to reduce their anxiety?
2   What help is available in the community to help the family cope with Mr Clements' period of hospitalization?

Following surgery, Mr Clements returns to the ward with an intravenous infusion in progress and a corrugated wound drain in situ.

3   Identify, giving reasons, the specific care required by Mr Clements in relation to the wound drain.
4   One potential problem of renal surgery is the development of a pneumothorax. Explain why this is so and identify how it would be recognized.
5   What would be the significance of your post-operative observations on Mr Clements' intake and output?
6   Outline the process by which surgical wounds heal.
7   What measures can the nursing staff take to ensure uncomplicated healing of Mr Clements' wound?
8   How would you evaluate the effectiveness of the above measures?

Mr Clements makes an excellent recovery and is ready for discharge 10 days after surgery.

9   What teaching will Mr Clements require in preparation for discharge?

4.2   Answers

1   Mr and Mrs Clements obviously fear that he will be incapacitated by the loss of a kidney. They should be reassured that the remaining kidney will be quite able to do the work of two kidneys without affecting his health. (This is assuming that his remaining kidney is healthy.) He may feel tired for some time following surgery but there is no reason for his life to be affected in any way. (The only things he should avoid are sports that might be dangerous and cause injury to the remaining kidney, e.g. rugby.)

2
*   Mr Clements will receive sickness benefit provided that he has been contributing to National Insurance Benefit.
*   There may be a local service providing transport to and from the hospital which is usually arranged by the Social Services Department.
*   A social worker may be able to provide care for the children while Mrs Clements visits her husband.
*   Possible voluntary organizations might offer help.
*   Help with fares may be available.

3   An open drainage system is used so that all drainage can be disposed of as quickly as possible. The drainage is likely to be serosanguineous fluid.

Nursing care	Reason
All dressings must be changed as soon as they become wet using an aseptic technique.	A wet dressing would be an ideal site for the multiplication of bacteria.
Apply a keyhole dressing around the drain and apply sterile padding.	This prevents too much drainage from coming into contact with the wound and allows the wound to drain freely. It also protects the skin.
Monitor the amount and type of drainage.	This gives an indication of the rate of healing or any infection.
Shorten the drain as directed.	This prevents pressure from the tubing on any part of the wound, which would cause tissue necrosis.
Remove the drain when directed by the surgeon.	When drainage has stopped the drain no longer fulfils any function.

Observe the site of drainage for 24 hours following removal. | This detects any undue drainage.

4   The kidneys are positioned in close proximity to the base of the lungs. This means that the diaphragmatic pleura may become accidentally perforated during the operation. This may result in the development of a pneumothorax which would manifest itself within 24 hours of surgery.

The following features should alert the nurse to the development of a pneumothorax:

- dyspnoea, tachypnoea
- sudden chest pain
- a feeling of extreme apprehension
- unequal chest expansion
- tachycardia, weak pulse
- low blood pressure
- pallor, dizziness

5   • Intravenous fluids must be monitored carefully to ensure that the correct fluid infuses at the correct rate.

- Alterations of the amount of fluid infused must be reported to the surgeon who will compensate for deficits/overloads.
- All urine output must be measured strictly every hour. Any evidence of abnormality such as reduced urine output may mean deterioration in the remaining kidney and must be reported immediately.
- Any vomit/nasogastric tube aspirate must be measured. A decreasing aspirate indicates a return of peristalsis. Excessive vomiting may lead to electrolyte imbalance.
- The passage of flatus should be noted as this is an indication that the intestines are regaining their function.
- Record the passage of faeces. If there is no bowel movement for more than 2 days after resumption of oral intake, Mr Clements may need an aperient.
- Observe the dietary intake when Mr Clements is back on oral intake. This gives an indication of his general condition.

6

Stage I—The wound is red, swollen and hot. Blood vessels breed and the platelets and fibrin cause clotting. Histamine released causes dilatation of capillary blood vessels. White blood cells enter the injured area resulting in oedema, increased colour and heat.
Stage II—Polymorphs and macrophages clear the wound of dead tissue.

Stage III—Fibroblasts continue to produce collagen. Vitamin C is essential for the production of collagen. Granulation tissue is formed. The wound is very fragile at this stage, so care must be taken during mobilization.

Stage IV—The scar tissue changes from pink to white. Collagen is produced for some months to strength the wound.

7
- Carry out aseptic technique, but only change the dressing when necessary.
- Practise thorough hand washing technique when attending to Mr Clements.
- Discourage Mr Clements from touching the wound.
- Provide fresh bed linen daily.
- Keep movement of dust to a minimum, e.g. during bed making.
- Discourage the patients from sitting on each other's beds.
- Ensure that Mr Clements gets sufficient rest and sleep.
- Provide Mr Clements with a nourishing diet which should be rich in protein (essential for tissue repair), contain vitamins A and C (for collagen synthesis) and contain minerals, particularly zinc (for enzyme activity).
- Promote circulation to ensure a sufficient supply of blood to the wound by:
  1 relieving undue pressure on the wound
  2 encouraging movement (with the help of a physiotherapist)

8 A concise description of the wound should be kept so that the progress of wound healing and the effectiveness of treatment can be evaluated. The condition of the suture line should be inspected and notes made concerning the presence of oedema, erythema, haematoma or any other abnormal conditions. Mr Clements' temperature should remain within normal limits and the wound should remain pink and uninflamed.

9 Mr Clements must attend for regular check-ups, when the remaining kidney will be checked for the development of further calculi.

He may need to be taught how to test his urine for the pH level. The reading that he should strive to maintain depends on the composition of the stone, as follows:

- **Uric acid stones** Mr Clements should maintain a relatively alkaline urine. This can be achieved by taking prescribed medication, e.g. sodium citrate.

- **Calcium/oxalate stones** Mr Clements should maintain a relatively acid urine. Acidifiers include vitamin C (ascorbic acid).

Dietary advice will again depend on the composition of the stone, as follows:

- **Fluid** He should drink a minimum of 2.5 litres of fluid a day to ensure a brisk flow of diluted urine through the kidneys.
- **Uric acid stones** Diet will be low in 'purine', so he should avoid liver, kidney, lean meat, whole grains, alcohol, dried beans, lentils, dried peas and spinach. He should also reduce those foods that produce an acid urine, e.g. plums, cheese, eggs.
- **Calcium stones** He should reduce those foods that are high in calcium, e.g. dairy produce.
- **Oxalate stones** He should avoid foods that are high in oxalate, e.g. rhubarb, spinach, asparagus, coffee, tea, strawberries.

Mr Clements should be told to consult his general practitioner if either of the following occur:

- chills, haematuria, loin pain
- sudden decrease in urinary output despite adequate intake. Mr Clements will be instructed as to when he can resume work and normal activities.

All this information should also be given in written form.

4.3   Miss Cotton—a young woman with nephrotic syndrome

Miss Cotton, a 28-year-old secretary, has been admitted to the ward with suspected nephrotic syndrome. She had gone to her general practitioner complaining of swollen ankles and eyelids. On routine urinalysis he found heavy proteinuria and referred her to the hospital for investigation and treatment.

On admission, Miss Cotton is noted to have a generalized pitting oedema and to be pale, extremely tired and lethargic. She is very concerned about her appearance and her weight gain.

1   With reference to Virginia Henderson's 'fundamental needs', what information would the nurse need to gather from Miss Cotton in order to plan her care?

A renal biopsy is booked, and in the meantime, treatment is commenced with prednisolone and spironolactone.

2   Identify the preparation Miss Cotton will require for the renal biopsy and the specific care she will require afterwards.

3   How can the accuracy of Miss Cotton's blood pressure reading be ensured?

4   Describe how you might teach a junior nurse to test Miss Cotton's urine.

5   With reference to normal and altered physiology explain why Miss Cotton will need a high protein/low salt diet.

6   From the following list of foods indicate those that she:
   (a) may take freely
   (b) may take in moderation
   (c) will not be allowed

- Tomatoes
- Potatoes
- Wholemeal bread
- Milk
- Cheese
- Eggs
- Tinned sardines
- Rice
- Fresh fish
- Steak
- Marmite
- Jam
- Syrup
- Butter
- Shredded Wheat
- Cocoa
- Fresh fruit juice
- Packet soups
- Bacon
- Fresh fruit
- Dry roasted peanuts
- Sausages

7 One of Miss Cotton's major problems is oedema. With reference to the actual/potential problems this may cause, identify the appropriate nursing actions that may be implemented.

Miss Cotton complains of feeling bored, especially as there are no other young patients on the ward.

8 What measures can the nursing staff take to alleviate Miss Cotton's boredom?

Eighteen days after her admission Miss Cotton has made a marked improvement. She has lost a total of 12 kg and is back to her normal weight. Her urinalysis shows that there is only slight proteinuria. She is to be discharged home having been prescribed prednisolone.

9 What information and advice will Miss Cotton require on discharge?

4.3   Answers

1

Fundamental needs	Information required
To breathe normally	Respiratory rate—as a base-line for further observations; any allergies, history of asthma, hay fever; any signs of pulmonary oedema.
To eat and drink adequately	Normal dietary intake; likes, dislikes, allergies, usual times of eating; weight; blood pressure.
To eliminate body wastes	Usual bowel and urinary habits; any recent changes in either.
To sleep and rest	Normal sleeping pattern; any problems with sleeping; level of exercise, activity tolerance.
To move and maintain a desirable position	Degree to which mobility is restricted by oedema.
To keep the body clean and well groomed	Normal hygiene routine, baths/showers; degree to which she will need to be assisted in carrying out bathing, hair washing, etc.
To communicate with others	Possible boyfriend, friends, parents, etc., who may be able to visit; phone number of next-of-kin; communication with employer.
To play/participate in forms of recreation	Hobbies, favourite pastimes; any preferences in reading matter; whether she has a radio she would like to bring in.
To worship according to one's faith	Any particular religious needs.

2   **Preparation**
   Miss Cotton should be given an explanation of what to expect during the biopsy and afterwards.
   - The doctor should measure the haemoglobin level, bleeding, clotting, prothrombin times and blood urea.
   - A plain X-ray will be done or an intravenous pyelogram to help accurately locate the kidney as a guide for needle insertion.

- Miss Cotton should be given instructions on the breathing pattern required during biopsy, i.e. taking several deep breaths, then holding a deep breath during inspiration.

Post-biopsy care
- Bed rest should be maintained for 24 hours.
- Pulse and blood pressure should be recorded half-hourly (or as hospital policy states) for 4 hours, then with decreasing frequency if stable. The nurse should monitor for signs of haemorrhage—a major complication which would be indicated by falling blood pressure, rapid pulse, and a dull, aching discomfort in the abdomen.
- All urine output should be observed for bleeding. Minor haematuria is common and should soon settle.

3
- Miss Cotton should be at rest during the reading.
- Measurements taken while the patient is lying down should always precede those taken while the patient is standing.
- A fairly quiet environment is required.
- Equipment should be in working order and the mercury tube must be cleaned regularly.
- The patient's arm should be held at the level of the heart.
- Ensure that the correct size cuff is used. It should cover no more than two-thirds of the upper arm, and the bladder should completely encircle the arm.
- Be aware of hospital policy for reading diastolic pressure, i.e. either at phase 4 or at phase 5. (Most doctors now agree that it should be read at phase 4.)

4
- Find out what she already knows and what she has been taught.
- Revise the normal physiology of passing urine and the normal constituents of urine.
- Demonstrate how to test Miss Cotton's urine. Discuss abnormal constituents of urine and their significance.
- Make use of visual aids, e.g. posters and diagrams, to aid your explanation.
- Allow the junior nurse to test urine under supervision.
- Give some extra reading references/homework.
- Test the nurse's knowledge with questions, a quiz, etc., after a period of time to allow for consolidation and practice.

5 Nephrotic syndrome is a collection of symptoms of underlying renal disease. The four characteristics are hypoproteinaemia, generalized oedema, proteinuria and hyperlipidaemia.

These characteristics may occur as a result of many other conditions or it may be idiopathic. Whatever the cause, the glomerular membrane becomes more permeable and allows plasma proteins through into the renal tubules. The protein that usually passes through the membrane is albumen, which is the smallest, but sometimes other larger plasma proteins follow. Albumen is mainly concerned with the maintenance of osmotic pressure at about 25 mmHg. With the loss of albumen the osmotic pressure falls and tissue fluid is not pulled back into the circulation. This leads to oedema. The resulting decrease in circulating volume causes retention of sodium and water under the influence of the renin–angiotensin mechanism. Miss Cotton will therefore need a high protein diet to replace lost proteins, and low salt to reduce aggravation of the oedema.

6

Foods that may be taken freely	Foods that may be taken in moderation	Foods that will not be allowed
Fresh fruit and juice	Wholemeal bread	Tinned sardines
Tomatoes	Milk	Marmite
Jam	Cheese	Syrup
Shredded Wheat	Eggs	Cocoa
Dry roasted peanuts	Fresh fish	Packet soups
Potatoes and rice (provided that they are cooked in non-salted water)	Butter	Bacon
		Sausages

7

Problem (actual/potential)	Nursing action
Difficulty in mobilizing	• Encourage bed rest but mobilization to the bathroom. • Ensure a comfortable position in bed.
Skin taut, shiny and fragile, and vulnerable to breakdown and infection	• Keep the skin clean and dry. • Encourage a daily shower with gentle drying, especially in the creases. • Instruct Miss Cotton to change position in bed 2-hourly. • Use sheepskins. • Keep the sheets clean and wrinkle free.

Cold extremities due to sluggish circulation	• Keep the limbs warm and encourage active exercises.
Anxiety about appearance	• Explain the cause of her swelling and treatment. • Explain how the weight will be lost and that normal appearance will be regained.
Anorexia	• Find out her likes and dislikes. • Provide small, frequent meals (and high protein drinks if she is not eating).

8   • Encourage Miss Cotton's boyfriend, friends and relatives to visit.
   • Ensure that she has access to a telephone.
   • Suggest that she brings in a personal stereo/radio if she has one.
   • Encourage her to continue with hobbies/interests. Introduce her to the library and mobile newspaper stall.
   • Spend time talking to Miss Cotton about her common interests.
   • When she is feeling better, involve her in the ward activities, e.g. helping with teas.

9   • How to test her urine for protein and an instruction to return if the tests show a large amount of protein
   • To return if her weight rises rapidly again
   • Advice and instructions regarding prednisolone therapy and a 'steroid card'
   • An instruction to take a 24-hour urine bottle so that she can bring a specimen with her to the outpatient department.
   • An explanation as to how she should collect the specimen.

4.4   Mr McCall—a man having a prostatectomy

Mr McCall, aged 65 years, is admitted to the ward at 8.30 p.m. with acute retention of urine. Mrs McCall had been concerned about his condition at home and had called the general practitioner who had immediately arranged for him to be admitted. Mrs McCall has remained at home, which is 20 miles away from the hospital.
Mr McCall has a 2-year history of difficulties with micturition but has resisted treatment until now. On admission he is extremely anxious about his condition and also about his wife.

Shortly after admission, catheterization is performed and gradual decompression of the bladder is commenced.

1   How might you reduce Mr McCall's anxiety level on admission to the ward?
2   With reference to normal and altered physiology how would you explain Mr McCall's condition to the junior nurse who has been assigned to work with you?
3   What observations should the nurse make of Mr McCall's urine output during decompression of the bladder and what would be the significance of these observations?

Following investigation the consultant decides to perform a transurethral prostatectomy 2 days later.

4   What pre-operative education will Mr McCall and his wife require?

As part of his pre-operative preparation Mr McCall is prescribed a premedication of papaveretum and hyoscine.

5   What actions should the nurse in charge take when she discovers an ampoule of the drug missing?

Mr McCall returns to the ward with an intravenous infusion in
progress and continuous bladder irrigation in situ to reduce the
possibility of clot formation in the bladder.

6   Why is haemorrhage a potential problem following this type
     of surgery and how would it be detected?
7   Another potential problem following surgery is the develop-
     ment of deep vein thrombosis. Giving reasons, what nurs-
     ing actions might be taken to prevent this and how would
     you recognize it should it develop?
8   Identify, giving reasons, the specific care required by
     Mr McCall in relation to his indwelling urinary catheter and
     bladder irrigation.

Three days following surgery the urinary catheter is removed.

9   What advice should be given to Mr McCall in order for him
     to regain urinary control?
10   What response would you make when Mr McCall asks if
     the operation will be likely to have any effect on his sex
     life?

4.4   Answers

1
- Explain all procedures beforehand, especially catheterization.
- Administer analgesia as prescribed.
- Encourage him to ask questions and spend time talking to him.
- Telephone his wife and keep her informed of his condition. Give him access to the phone and ensure privacy.

2   Draw a diagram to show the position of the prostate gland. The prostate gland secretes a thin milky-looking alkaline solution which reduces the acidity of seminal fluid and vaginal secretions. Sperm are more mobile in a neutral or slightly alkaline medium.

After the age of 40 years, the prostate gland in nearly all men begins to hypertrophy and enlarge. The exact cause of this is unknown. In 1 in 10 of men the prostate gland becomes so enlarged as to cause obstruction to the outflow of urine from the bladder. The bladder muscle, in an attempt to overcome the obstruction, hypertrophies. Gradually, the bladder becomes less able to empty itself of urine. Residual urine increases, leading to chronic retention. Occasionally the bladder muscles fail suddenly as in Mr McCall's case and causes acute retention of urine.

3   The nurse should monitor the amount of urine being released from the bladder and observe for blood in the urine. A sudden release of urine could precipitate haemorrhage. Sudden filling of small blood vessels previously constricted in the bladder mucosa may cause rupture.

4
- Give Mr McCall an explanation regarding the need for surgery and the type of surgery to be performed. Emphasize that there will be no visible scar.
- Tell him what to expect post-operatively, i.e. intravenous infusion, urinary catheterization and continuous bladder irrigation. For how long is he likely to have these?
- Teach him deep breathing and leg exercises. Teach Mrs McCall these exercises also so that she may encourage him to cooperate.
- Tell him how long he is likely to be in hospital.
- Warn him that urine is expected to be tinged with blood in the early post-operative period.
- Advise him how to cope with the urge to void caused by the presence of the indwelling urinary catheter.

5   Papaveretum is a drug controlled under the Misuse of Drugs

Act (1971) which governs its supply, storage and prescription. All stocks of the drug must be accounted for in the record book. The nurse in charge should take the following actions:

- Recheck the number of ampoules in the cupboard with a second nurse.
- Check with other staff nurses on the ward and check all drug charts.
- If the error is still not accounted for, report the incident to the senior nurse (Nursing Officer) and to the pharmacist. If the missing ampoule is not found the police may be informed.

6 The prostate gland is highly vascular. During the surgery the area is continuously irrigated to wash away debris and blood. The pressure of the irrigating fluid is sufficient to temporarily stop any bleeding from open veins. The open vein may therefore not be identified and coagulated. Once irrigation stops, bleeding begins again.

Mr McCall should be monitored for increasing pulse rate, decreasing blood pressure, pallor, feelings of apprehension, and bright red drainage from the catheter, all of which may indicate haemorrhage.

7

Nursing action	Rationale
Pre-operatively, educate Mr McCall regarding post-operative mobility and exercises.	Prior knowledge increases cooperation post-operatively.
Encourage Mr McCall to change his position frequently while he is in bed and to carry out leg exercises.	This improves venous return and reduces pooling in the veins.
Discourage Mr McCall from crossing his legs or sitting with his knees flexed while in bed.	This may impede venous return. Sitting with the knees flexed encourages pooling of blood in the deep veins of the calf.
Use antiembolic stockings if prescribed. These must be removed at least daily to enable skin care to be carried out.	Stockings reduce venous stasis.

Keep them free from wrinkles and rolls.	Rolled stockings may impede circulation.
Assist Mr McCall out of bed (after consulting the surgeon).	Moving about improves circulation and venous return.

Deep vein thrombosis is a 'silent' process. Generally there are no evident signs or symptoms. The patient may complain of tenderness in the calf and there may be swelling and/or redness of the affected area.

8
- Perform catheter toilet (according to hospital policy). This helps to keep the catheter exit site free from exudate and reduces the incidence of infection.
- Maintain a closed system of drainage. Use the distal emptying outlet to empty the bag. A closed system is effective in reducing infection.
- 'Milk' the drainage tubing frequently and prevent kinking or obstruction of the tubing in order to maintain an unobstructed flow at all times.
- Regulate the rate of bladder irrigation according to the degree of haematuria. If drainage is bright red, infuse rapidly. As drainage clears (which should occur within 24 hours of surgery) slow down the rate of irrigation. The purpose of the continuous irrigation is to remove blood from the bladder before it has time to clot and obstruct the bladder and catheter.
- Maintain an accurate fluid intake and output chart and irrigation chart. This enables any renal dysfunction to be detected early.
- Encourage Mr McCall to drink at least 3 litres of fluid in 24 hours. This helps to flush out the catheter.
- Wash hands thoroughly before and after attending to Mr McCall's catheter. This prevents cross-infection.

9
- Explain that dribbling and incontinence are not uncommon following prostatectomy but that this is temporary.
- Reassure him that a burning sensation is common following removal of a catheter for about 24 hours.
- Teach perineal exercises. While standing, tighten and relax the gluteal muscles five times each hour. This facilitates the return of adequate sphincter control. While voiding, Mr McCall should voluntarily stop and restart urinary stream using the sphincter muscles. He should lengthen the time between each voiding by consciously holding his urine.
- Suggest that he avoids tea and coffee. These contain caffeine, which is a mild diuretic.

10 His ability to have an erection is unaffected; therefore there
will be no change in his ability to have sex.

However, the passage of semen may be affected. Following surgery, semen may flow into the bladder rather than
through the penis. If this happens his urine may appear
cloudy after intercourse. This is completely normal and
should not give cause for concern.

A time lapse of about 6–8 weeks should elapse between
surgery and the resumption of intercourse, though the doctor will tell him when sex can be resumed. This time interval
allows for healing of the internal wound.

4.5 Mrs Semple—an elderly woman with incontinence

During your community experience you accompany the community nurse to visit Mrs Martha Semple, aged 70 years, who lives alone in a two-bedroomed house. She has been widowed for 4 years. She has two children, both of whom are married with families of their own. They both live some distance away from Mrs Semple.

Over the past few months Mrs Semple has become increasingly isolated in her house and very rarely goes out. She has painful feet and suffers from arthritis, and is therefore finding it difficult to walk too far.

One of Mrs Semple's major problems is incontinence. There is a strong smell of urine in the house and she is very obviously deeply ashamed of her problem.

1 Identify the factors which may be contributing to Mrs Semple's incontinence and which would be investigated during assessment.
2 With reference to normal and altered physiology explain micturition and describe the various types of incontinence and their causes.

As part of her assessment Mrs Semple is asked to keep a chart to show how often she is passing urine and how often she is wet.

3 What significant information can be gained from such a chart?

Following assessment several problems are identified which may be contributing to the major problem of incontinence. These are:
• depression and lack of motivation
• loneliness
• difficulty in walking due to arthritis and overgrown toe-nails

4 List the members of the community health care team who may become involved in solving Mrs Semple's problems.

5   What actions may be taken to try to overcome the three problems identified above?

In order to try to reduce incontinence a toilet training programme is introduced.

6   What are the principles of such a programme?
7   What aids are available for Mrs Semple to use until she has regained more control over her bladder?
8   How might the effectiveness of Mrs Semple's management best be evaluated after 3 months?

4.5   Answers

1   • **Physical factors** Possible urinary tract infections; the effect of ageing (a gradual decline in tone of muscles, a degree of uterine–urethral prolapse, atrophic changes and vaginal irritations caused by hormonal changes, the feeling that incontinence is normal in the elderly); visual disability; painful feet and difficulty in walking; slowness in moving.
   • **Environment factors** The location of the toilet (may have difficulty reaching it in time); whether the toilet is warm; low chairs may prevent Mrs Semple from getting up quickly enough.
   • **Confusion** Depression of the mental ability to recognize bladder distension. Drugs, e.g. tranquillizers and sedatives, may depress mental functions.
   • **Psychological/emotional factors** Depression; attention-seeking personality; reactions of society towards incontinence; loneliness; feelings of rejection and uselessness; bereavement.
   • **Diet and fluid intake** Obesity; constipation; dehydration.

2   Micturition occurs when the muscular wall of the bladder contracts and the internal and external sphincters open. The muscles of the internal sphincter are smooth fibres and are not under the control of the will; those of the external sphincter are striated muscle and are under voluntary control.

   Micturition is controlled by the nervous system. The accumulation of urine in the bladder stimulates stretch receptors in the bladder wall. Impulses pass along sensory fibres of pelvic nerves to the spinal cord and are transmitted back to the muscle of the bladder via the parasympathetic fibres. This is the micturition reflex, which causes contraction of the muscular wall of the bladder. With this muscular contraction the internal sphincter is pulled open. In babies, this reflex will result in micturition. In an adult however, the reflex can be inhibited by higher centres in the cortex until it is convenient to pass urine.

   Incontinence means passing urine at the wrong time in the wrong place. The types of incontinence are:
   • **true/total incontinence** caused by injury or neurogenic disease, leading to changes in nervous innovation
   • **stress incontinence** caused by inefficient pelvic muscles
   • **'urge incontinence'**, which has various causes including

infection, bladder tumours, upper motor neurone lesion and psychological problems
- **overflow incontinence** caused by obstructive disorders of the bladder, urinary retention following surgery, and injury to the spine at the sacral level

3 Frequency of micturition
- Number of incontinent episodes
- When the incontinent episodes occur
- Whether sleep is disturbed by micturition
- The capacity of the bladder if the volume is also measured. This type of chart can also help the doctor to identify the type of incontinence.

4
- General practitioner
- Health visitor
- Continence adviser
- Physiotherapist
- Chiropodist
- Social worker

5 **Problem—depression and lack of motivation**
- Set achievable goals to give Mrs Semple something to aim for.
- Spend time talking to Mrs Semple to find out about her problems, worries, etc.
- Involve the social worker in helping with any financial/housing problems.
- Involve Mrs Semple's family, especially her grandchildren.
- Arrange for Mrs Semple to attend a local centre for physiotherapy.
- Ensure that Mrs Semple is sleeping well enough.

Problem—loneliness
- Encourage the family to visit frequently and bring grandchildren.
- Arrange for Mrs Semple to attend a day centre, which will introduce her to new people.
- Encourage Mrs Semple to join a local group.
- Arrange a visit from the local vicar. Local schools may run schemes to visit the elderly.
- Help her to regain urinary control, which will boost her confidence and enable her to venture out more.

Problem—difficulty in walking due to arthritis and overgrown toe-nails
- Arrange an appointment wih a chiropodist.
- Arrange visits to a physiotherapist, who will teach her exercises and enable her to become more active.

     • Organize transport to take her to appointments initially.

6   The aim of a toileting programme is to promote continence. The programme is based on the information gained in the frequency chart and is therefore tailored to suit the individual. Toileting times are worked out to anticipate likely need. This may result in visits to the toilet at regular intervals during the day or at variable intervals. The programme is evaluated after 4 or 5 days and readjusted as necessary.

     Some forms of toileting programmes aim to retrain the bladder by encouraging the individual to extend the time interval between visits to the toilet. This results in an increase in bladder capacity.

7   The aids that Mrs Semple is introduced to will be assessed on individual needs, but the following are available:
- Incontinence pads and pants. Pads come in a variety of sizes, thickness and shapes.
- Bed protection—bed pads, disposable drawsheets, washable absorbable sheets, plastic mattress covers.
- Commode, hand-held urinals—if unable to reach the toilet in time.
- Adapted clothing, deodorants.

8
- Examine the frequency chart. This should show a reduction in the number of times she is incontinent.
- Assess the ability to dispense with any aids she has been using, e.g. commode, pads, etc.
- Find out how much she is going out, whether she has made new friends, and whether she feels less depressed.
- Find out how often she sees her family.

4.6   Mrs Westley—a woman with acute renal failure

Mrs Rachael Westley, aged 35 years, has been admitted to hospital
with multiple fractures following a road traffic accident. Six hours after
admission it is noted that Mrs Westley has not yet passed urine. Acute
renal failure is diagnosed following blood investigation.

1   Identify the observations the nurse should make on Mrs
    Westley that are specific to her renal failure, and with refer-
    ence to altered physiology explain their significance.
2   Outline the dietary management Mrs Westley will require
    during the oliguric stage.
3   From the following list identify those foods that are high in
    protein and which therefore are restricted:

- Mushrooms
- Lentils
- Cauliflower (boiled)
- Watercress
- Peaches (fresh)
- Bananas
- Prunes
- Peas
- Malt bread
- Plums
- Instant coffee
- Tangerines
- Chocolate
- Celery (boiled)
- Strawberries
- Rhubarb
- Apples
- Nuts

Conservative management continues until tests reveal rising blood urea
and potassium levels. Peritoneal dialysis is commenced.

4   With reference to anatomy and physiology explain the prin-
    ciples of dialysis.
5   Giving reasons identify the specific care Mrs Westley will
    require during peritoneal dialysis.
6   Draw up a care plan to show how the nurse might cope
    with those problems associated with the body's attempt to
    excrete urea via the skin and mucous membranes.

Mr Westley visits his wife frequently and participates in her care. He is obviously concerned and anxious about his wife and enquires about her future prognosis.

7 How might the nurse respond to Mr Westley's questions?

Eighteen days following the onset of acute renal failure, Mrs Westley begins to pass increasing amounts of dilute urine. Mrs Westley's fluid intake is gradually increased, as is the amount of protein in her diet. The doctor orders a 24-hour urine collection for creatinine clearance.

8 Describe the nurse's role in the collection of the 24-hour urine specimen.
9 How would you explain to a junior nurse the significance of a creatinine clearance?

4.6   Answers

1

Observation	Significance	Altered physiology
Respirations	Increasing dyspnoea may indicate pulmonary oedema. Deep, rapid respirations may indicate acidosis. 'Uraemic odour' presents in advanced renal failure.	Failure to excrete sodium and water expands the extracellular fluid compartment. Failure to excrete H^+ ions leads to a fall in pH (acidosis) and an attempt to excrete urea.
Pulse	A weak, rapid pulse may be indicative of heart failure. A slow, irregular pulse is a sign of hyperkalaemia.	Heart failure is precipitated by overhydration. Serum potassium rises as it is liberated from cells in tissue breakdown, and cannot be excreted.
Blood pressure	A progressive rise in blood pressure may indicate increasing uraemia.	An increase in blood volume occurs as a result of retention of sodium and water and secretion of renin.
Temperature	Pyrexia is indicative of infection.	Pyrexia results from suppression of the immune system.
Weight (daily)	No loss or gain in weight usually indicates fluid retention.	Expanded extra-cellular fluid compart-ment leads to oedema and weight gain.
Fluid intake and output chart	An output of less than 30 ml hourly or 500 ml daily is ominous. Increasing output indicates diuresis and returning renal function.	Reduced renal perfusion leads to renal ischaemia and reduced glomerular filtration rate (GFR).
	Input must be restricted at the oliguric stage.	The diuretic stage occurs when GFR rises.

General behaviour for evidence of twitching, drowsiness, disorientation and headache	This is indicative of uraemia, cerebral oedema, approaching convulsions and coma.	An inability of the kidney to excrete metabolic waste products leads to a build-up of toxic materials in the blood.

2   Daily fluid intake must be limited to 500 ml plus a volume equal to the urinary output of the previous 24 hours. The 500 ml replaces insensible losses from faeces, sweat and respirations. Fluids must be low in protein and electrolytes but high in carbohydrate to prevent the breakdown of body protein for energy. Hycal and Caloreen are examples of suitable high energy glucose additives for drinks.

3   • Mushrooms
    • Lentils
    • Watercress
    • Bananas
    • Prunes
    • Malt bread
    • Instant coffee
    • Chocolate
    • Rhubarb
    • Nuts

4   Dialysis refers to the separation of two solutions by a semi-permeable membrane through which some solutes and water may pass. The size of the pores in the dialysis membranes ensures that only small molecules pass through, and not proteins and blood cells. Water passes from the area of lower osmotic pressure to that of greater osmotic pressure. Molecules pass from an area of higher concentration to one of lower concentration.

In peritoneal dialysis the semi-permeable membrane is the peritoneum which separates the dialysis fluid from the patient's interstitial fluid.

Substances removed during dialysis are water, electrolytes, urea, creatinine, and uric acid in concentrations regulated by the type of dialysis fluid used.

5

Nursing care	Reasons
Explain peritoneal dialysis.	This reduces anxiety, increases cooperation and enhances recovery. Allow for verbalization of fears.
Weigh daily. (Preferably nurse on a weigh bed.)	This is helpful in assessing the state of hydration by measuring daily fluctuations in weight.
Keep an exact record of fluid balance and timing of exchanges.	If not all fluid is recovered Mrs Westley may develop circulatory overload.
Take 4-hourly temperature readings.	This detects any infection.
Monitor respirations, blood pressure and pulse.	A drop in blood pressure may indicate excessive fluid loss. Alterations in the pulse may indicate impending shock. 　　Respiratory difficulty may be caused by upward pressure from fluid in the peritoneal cavity.
Promote Mrs Westley's comfort by regular movement.	The dialysis period is lengthy and she may become uncomfortable in one position.

6

Problem	Goal	Nursing Action
Disagreeable taste in mouth	For Mrs Westley to have a fresh mouth	• Pleasant-tasting toothpaste • Lemon drops to suck • Ice cubes
Stomatitis	For Mrs Westley's mouth to remain healthy	• Regular teeth cleaning • Mouthwashes • Petroleum jelly for the lips

Potential pressure sores	For Mrs Westley's skin to remain healthy and intact	• Turned at regular intervals • Use of sheepskins • Skin hygiene • Crease-free bed linen
Pruritus	For Mrs Westley to be comfortable	• Daily bath

7   The nurse should first find out what Mr Westley already knows about his wife's condition and what he has been told. If the nurse is unsure of what to say she should enlist the help of the sister/doctor immediately and not delay answering. She can explain what has happened and the effects of acute renal failure. In most instances, acute renal failure is reversible, but Mrs Westley may take some time to show any signs of recovery. Long-term prognosis, if she recovers, is excellent.

8   Mrs Westley should be kept at rest during the test as creatinine is produced during muscular activity. When the collection is started, the first specimen is discarded. At the end of the 24 hours Mrs Westley should be asked to void and this is included in the specimen. The specimen should be kept cool. Mrs Westley must be given instructions regarding the test.

9   A creatinine clearance test includes a 24-hour urine collection and a venous blood specimen. From the urine collection the rate of urinary excretion of creatinine per minute is calculated. Normal in the adult is about 1.2–1.7 g per 24 hours.

From the blood specimen the volume of plasma cleared of creatinine per minute (the glomerular filtration rate) is calculated.

The creatinine clearance test therefore gives an indication of renal function.

5 Care of the Patient Approaching Death

5.1   Mr Stanton—an elderly man in the terminal stages of carcinoma of the bronchus

Mr Stanton, aged 72 years, has inoperable carcinoma of the bronchus which was diagnosed 7 months ago. Since he was discharged from hospital Mr Stanton has been looked after at home by his 66-year-old wife and her two married daughters who live close by. The family wish to continue to care for Mr Stanton at home, even though he needs constant attention.

Before Mr Stanton was discharged from hospital the district sister carried out a home assessment.

1   What information would have been collected during this first assessment?
2   List the members of the primary health care team who may be involved in Mr Stanton's care and management at home.

Mr Stanton's condition deteriorates fairly rapidly and he is now dyspnoeic, extremely thin, and confined to bed. He is occasionally incontinent of urine.

3   What equipment is available to facilitate home nursing and how can the family obtain this equipment?
4   How can Mrs Stanton be helped to:
   (a) make breathing easier for her husband?
   (b) keep his skin clean and healthy?

Mr Stanton's pain is controlled by the administration of oral diamorphine every 4 hours.

5   Identify the factors that may lower Mr Stanton's pain threshold and those that may raise his pain threshold.
6   With reference to the factors identified above identify the

measures other than medication that can be implemented to relieve Mr Stanton's pain and discomfort.

7   How can the family be helped to cope with the stress of caring for Mr Stanton?

During a conversation with the district sister, Mrs Stanton admits to being frightened of what to expect when her husband dies.

---

8   What reassurance can the nurse give Mrs Stanton in order to help her cope with her husband's impending death?

Mr Stanton dies peacefully in his own home 8 months after diagnosis. His wife is with him.

---

9   What practical help is available to help Mrs Stanton and the family with funeral arrangements?
10 Identify the stages of reaction to loss that Mrs Stanton may pass through, and the support available to help her cope with bereavement.

5.1 Answers

1 Information can be gathered by asking the following questions:
   - What facilities are available? Is the bedroom upstairs? Can the bed be moved downstairs? Is there enough room to move about? Where is the toilet? How can the family be helped to provide a restful atmosphere?
   - How able is Mrs Stanton to cope with household activities and how much will the family be involved?
   - What is the emotional state of Mrs Stanton and the family?
   - What equipment/help might the family need in the initial stages?
   - What do the family understand about Mr Stanton's condition and the effects it will have on him?

2 - General practitioner
   - District nurse
   - Social worker
   - Nurse from the Macmillan Service *or* the Marie Curie Foundation
   - Physiotherapist
   - Occupational therapist
   - Home help

3 - Ripple mattresses; bedcradles; commode; bedpan; Zimmer frame; wheelchair; feeding utensils; incontinence pads/sheeting.
   - Draw mackintosh, draw sheets, laundry service.
   - Condom drainage if Mr Stanton is incontinent.
   - Extra pillows—Mr Stanton will need support in bed.
   - Minor adaptations, e.g. bath rails, stair rails.

   Mrs Stanton can gain any of the above equipment by approaching the district nurse or social worker. If the person they approach cannot get the equipment they will put them in touch with the people who can.

4 (a) **Breathing**
   - Explain and demonstrate how to support Mr Stanton in a sitting position by the use of a back rest or armchair.
   - Reduce fear and anxiety by ensuring that he is not left alone. Administer medication as prescribed.
   - Help Mrs Stanton to give steam inhalations if he has a cough. Involve the physiotherapist.
   - Explain about the importance of fresh air. Oxygen can be provided.

(b) **Skin**
Show Mrs Stanton how to inspect the skin and how to recognize problems.

The district nurse should visit daily to give Mr Stanton a bed bath. (She may visit more frequently as his condition deteriorates.) Mrs Stanton can give him washes during the day as required.

Mr Stanton should be encouraged to sit out of bed as much as he is able. When he is eventually confined to bed he needs to be turned regularly. The family can help to move him and the nurses should visit at regular intervals.

Mr Stanton can be provided with urinals/condom drainage. Mrs Stanton should be instructed how to use these to prevent incontinence.

Equipment as mentioned in ans. 3 can help to facilitate nursing care.

The nurses attending Mr Stanton should constantly assess and evaluate the care being given. A nursing care plan should be drawn up with Mrs Stanton's involvement and a copy left in the house.

5 Factors that may lower the pain threshold include:
  - anxiety
  - fear
  - insomnia
  - anger
  - discomfort
  - tiredness
  - sadness
  - depression

Factors that may raise the pain threshold include:
  - Sleep and rest
  - Relief of nausea and vomiting
  - Sympathy
  - Diversion therapy
  - Understanding
  - Contact with close relatives and company

6 Arrange for somebody to be with Mr Stanton. Involve the family. Physical discomfort can be reduced by the presence of an understanding person. Mr Stanton may also find he can talk to a companion, thereby relieving some of his fears and anxieties. The following measures can also be used to relieve Mr Stanton's pain and discomfort:
  - Ensure that Mr Stanton is in a comfortable position.
  - Maintain his skin in a healthy condition. This reduces discomfort.

- Encourage relaxation, deep breathing and soft, relaxing music.
- Use diversional therapy.
- Use heat and cold applications and massage.
- Facilitate sleep and rest, a quiet environment, comfort, hot drinks and talk.
- If suitable, involve clergy.

7   The involvement of members of the primary health care team as listed in ans. 2 can relieve the stress of having to attend to Mr Stanton continually.

A home help and Meals-on-Wheels reduce the amount of work Mrs Stanton has to do and allows her to spend time with her husband.

Give relevant telephone numbers to Mrs Stanton so that she can get help whenever necessary.

The district nurse should check that Mrs Stanton is getting sufficient food, sleep and rest herself. The general practitioner may prescribe some sedatives for her.

Give Mrs Stanton time to go out while the nurses stay with her husband.

Give time for the family to talk about their feelings and fears to, for example, a social worker or clergyman.

Provide help with all nursing care.

Local volunteer agencies may provide company for Mr Stanton enabling Mrs Stanton to have a break from the house.

Financial assistance may reduce some of the burden of caring for Mr Stanton.

8   Explain how to recognize impending death. Reassure Mrs Stanton that she can ring for the nurse at any time. Check she has the correct telephone number.

Reassure her that Mr Stanton's death is liable to be peaceful and that he will be maintained pain free. She may be frightened of how he might die, so any misconceptions must be sorted out.

Encourage her daughters to stay with her towards the end. Mrs Stanton should ideally not be left alone with her husband.

Talk to Mrs Stanton about her fears to ascertain any particular ones she may have. Encourage her to talk about her husband.

9   The undertaker will be contacted; often the nurse may offer to contact him. He will explain what has to be done and will support the family through the funeral.

Financial help is available and a social worker can give

practical advice on dealing with mortgage, allowances, pensions, etc.

10
- Denial
- Anger
- Depression
- Bargaining
- Acceptance   (Kubler-Ross, 1970)

The social worker may often visit the family after the death to talk to the bereaved and support them. Bereavement counselling may be available. 'Cruse' is a national organization for widows/widowers. Many hospitals run bereavement discussion groups. A chaplain may be able to visit Mrs Stanton.

5.2   Mr Goldsmith—an adult dying from leukaemia

Mr Joseph Goldsmith, aged 58 years, has chronic lymphoblastic
leukaemia. His condition was diagnosed 3½ years ago and since then
has had intermittent chemotherapy and radiotherapy. Two months ago
Mr Goldsmith's blood picture indicated relapse, and further vigorous
treatment was initiated. However, therapy failed to bring about any
improvement and eventually, following discussion with Mr and
Mrs Goldsmith, all treatment was discontinued. Until now
Mr Goldsmith's family have been caring for him at home. This has
become very difficult for them and Mrs Goldsmith no longer feels able
to cope. Mr Goldsmith has therefore been admitted to the ward for
terminal care. On admission, Mr Goldsmith, who is an Orthodox Jew,
is noted to be extremely thin, and is unable to get out of bed. His
mouth is sore and his gums ulcerated and bleeding, and he has very
little appetite. He has been having regular analgesia at home but his
wife is worried that he is still in considerable pain.

1   Discuss the steps the nurse can take to establish effective
    communication with Mr Goldsmith and his wife on admis-
    sion.
2   How can the nurse assess Mr Goldsmith's pain on admis-
    sion?
3   Describe the nursing actions that may be implemented to
    promote a clean and comfortable mouth.
4   What steps can the nurse take to ensure that Mr Goldsmith
    maintains his nutritional intake?
5   With reference to normal and altered physiology what
    would you tell a junior nurse about the effects of chronic
    lymphoblastic leukaemia?

Mr Goldsmith has been in hospital for 3 days when, during
conversation, he admits to the nurse that he is very frightened of
dying.

6   Identify Mr Goldsmith's possible fears and discuss how the
    nurse can best help to allay these fears.

With good nursing care and support from nursing staff and his wife, Mr Goldsmith remains fairly comfortable. However, his condition continues to deteriorate slowly over the next 2 weeks.

7 What changes may the nurse observe in Mr Goldsmith that indicate impending death?

Mr Goldsmith dies peacefully 3 weeks after his admission with his wife and children by his side.

8 What should the nurse know (or be able to find out) about Mr Goldsmith's faith in order to carry out appropriate care after his death?
9 What knowledge should the nurse have regarding the legal aspects associated with:
   (a) the disposal of Mr Goldsmith's personal belongings?
   (b) the death certificate?
10 How can the staff on the ward be helped to come to terms with Mr Goldsmith's death?

5.2 Answers

1 Ashworth (*Communicate to care*, RCN, 1980) refers to the positive effects of physical proximity, eye contact, friendly tone, and conversation regarding personal topics. So when trying to establish relationships, take notice of the following points:

- Sit close to Mr Goldsmith so that it is easy to talk face to face.
- Greet Mr and Mrs Goldsmith in a friendly manner, and smile.
- Address Mr Goldsmith by his correct title and show warmth of tone.
- Utilize touch. Take Mr Goldsmith's hand in initial greeting and do not hestitate to hold his hand gently if appropriate.
- Do not hurry the initial meeting.
- Only ask the minimum of necessary questions initially to avoid overtiring him.
- The nurse should try to come to terms with her own attitudes towards death and dying.
- Find out from Mrs Goldsmith how much Mr Goldsmith knows about his condition in order to avoid misunderstandings.
- Create a pleasing, happy environment.

2
- Observe Mr Goldsmith's facial expression and posture.
- Talk to Mr Goldsmith and also to his wife to ascertain:
  1 when he notices the pain
  2 how he relieves the pain
  3 what seems to trigger the pain
  4 how he reacts to pain
  5 whether the pain makes him fearful/anxious
  6 whether he expects to be pain free
  7 where the pain is (use a body chart to record the sites of pain). Ask him to describe his pain and whether it varies during the day.
- Ascertain the dosage and name of the drug he is on at that time and how often he is taking it.

3
- Encourage as much self-help as possible.
- Use a small, soft toothbrush to remove debris from the teeth. An electric toothbrush may be helpful.
- Use foam sticks and a swabbed finger if a toothbrush is too abrasive.
- Use solutions (sodium bicarbonate, hydrogen peroxide

3%) when necessary to remove mucus and crusts. Vitamin C tablets may be dissolved on the tongue.

- Use mouthwashes, e.g. Corsodyl, Redoxon. Normal saline, fruit juices, lemon juice and chewing gum stimulate the salivary glands.
- Keep his lips moist and soft with K-Y lubricating jelly or Vaseline.
- Encourage intake of fluids.
- Inspect Mr Goldsmith's mouth daily using a pen torch.
- Report any abnormalities, e.g. *Candida* infections, so that treatment can be commenced.

4   All Mr Goldsmith's food and drink must be kosher (i.e. the animals must be slaughtered in a special way) and food from the pig is forbidden. He must not have milk and meat at the same meal. Mr Goldsmith may ask to wash his hands and say a blessing before he eats.

It is important for the nurse to take these factors into account when trying to meet Mr Goldsmith's nutritional needs. The following steps can also be taken:

- Control any distressing symptoms that cause anorexia, e.g. pain, nausea and vomiting.
- Administer mouth care as in ans. **3**.
- Administer appetite stimulants if ordered.
- Find out Mr Goldsmith's likes and dislikes and encourage Mrs Goldsmith to bring in anything he particularly fancies.
- Provide him with small, attractive meals and give him time to eat.
- Offer nourishing fluids when Mr Goldsmith cannot eat.
- Give assistance to Mr Goldsmith if he needs it.
- Encourage a fluid intake of 1 litre/24 hours but realize that he will only take sips of water as he deteriorates.

5   • **Normal physiology** All blood cells develop from one common cell—the reticuloendothelial cell in the lymph and bone marrow.

All cells go through a series of changes from a reticuloendothelial cell to their mature/adult form.

White cells are divided into two main classes: granulocytes and agranulocytes.

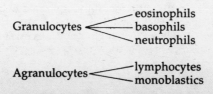

Functions of the various blood cells are as follows:
1 **Erythrocytes**—carriage of oxygen and carbon dioxide
2 **Granulocytes**—phagocytosis
3 **Agranulocytes**—immunity
4 **Platelets**—blood clotting

- **Altered physiology** Leukaemia is a condition in which there is an excessive, uncontrolled production of white blood cells in their immature 'blast' form. In lymphoblastic leukaemia, there is a proliferation of lymphoblasts. Because the cells are immature they cannot fulfil their normal function. Because of an overproduction of lymphoblasts the production of all other blood cells in the bone marrow is reduced, giving rise to the following pathological changes:
  1 anaemia—lethargy, pallor, dyspnoea on exertion
  2 bleeding tendencies, bruising, epistaxis
  3 reduced resistance to infection
  4 marrow hyperplasia, pain
  5 enlargement of the spleen and lymph nodes

6
- Fear of a painful, agonizing death
- Fear of losing control and becoming dependent on others
- Worry about what will happen to his family
- Fear of separation from his family, friends and job
- Fear of failing to fulfil obligations or a life task
- Fear of death as a punishment
- Fear of a lonely death
- Fear of what will happen to him after death

It is important for the nurse to respond to Mr Goldsmith's fears. If the fear is unrealistic he must be given reassurance and explanations. If it is realistic, the nurse must help the patient to cope with the losses and grief. The nurse can help to overcome the above fears by:

- reassuring Mr Goldsmith that the moment of death from leukaemia is very likely to be peaceful and that he will be given drugs to maintain his pain relief.
- showing an interest in Mr Goldsmith, listening to what he has to say, and reassuring him that his family will be able to cope on their own.
- encouraging family members and close friends to visit. No restrictions should be placed upon times of visiting.
- helping Mr Goldsmith to look at the positive aspects of his life.
- providing time for Mr Goldsmith to practise his religious

obligations. Friends and relatives may feel a religious duty to visit.

- contacting the Rabbi and informing him of Mr Goldsmith's condition.

7
- He may become restless, agitated and uncomfortable and he may begin plucking at the sheets.
- He may lose interest in what is going on around him.
- He may become less willing to take food and fluid. His mouth will become dry.
- He may become extremely pale, cyanosed and jaundiced.
- His pulse will become weak, rapid, thready and irregular. It may have to be felt at the carotid artery or at the apex of the heart.
- Breathing may alter. Noisy breathing—'the death rattle'—is due to the accumulation of secretions that he is too weak to cough up. He may also suffer from Cheyne–Stokes respiration or hiccups.
- He may be incontinent of urine/faeces. Retention may occur, making him restless.
- His body will become increasingly cold to the touch.
- He may lapse into a coma preceding death.

8
- Leave his body untouched for 8 minutes to 1½ hours.
- Allow his eldest son to close his eyes and mouth.
- Wear gloves when handling the body. The nurse is only permitted to close his eyes, straighten the limbs and bind the jaw. A Gentile must not defile the body.
- Empty any water in the vicinity of the bed.
- Cover any mirrors in Mr Goldsmith's room.
- Cover the body with a sheet and place a candle close to his head.
- Be aware that handling the body by a Jewish person on the Sabbath is forbidden.
- The body will be transferred to the mortuary where the Rabbi or member of the family will be in attendance.
- Orthodox Jews do not allow autopsies.
- The nurse can ask the Rabbi if she does not know what to do, or she may follow hospital procedure.

9
(a) Any valuables should have already been locked in the safe and these can be collected by Mrs Goldsmith when convenient. All other belongings should be listed by two nurses who must both sign the list as a correct record. The property will be packed and given to Mrs Goldsmith at a suitable time.

(b) Mr Goldsmith's doctor will sign the death certificate.

This certificate will be given to Mrs Goldsmith. The death must be registered as soon as possible. Mrs Goldsmith should be given instructions about where to take the certificate.

10
- Information about Mr Goldsmith and his death must be shared with all members of staff.
- Senior nurses must be aware of those nurses who may have become closely involved in his care.
- Staff must be given an opportunity to talk about their feelings as soon after his death as possible.
- It may be useful to have the clinical psychologist at the meeting.
- There should be somewhere on the ward for staff to find some privacy and have a break from the ward.
- It may help some of the nurses to cope by attending Mr Goldsmith's funeral.

5.3 Mr Robinson—a man with liver failure

Mr Mathew Robinson, aged 48 years, has been in hospital for 2 weeks during which time the diagnosis of advanced liver failure due to cirrhosis has been confirmed.

Mr Robinson has been an alcoholic for many years but, despite therapy, still continues to drink alcohol. He is single and has one sister who lives abroad and with whom he has not kept in touch.

1 Discuss how Mr Robinson might react over the next few weeks after the doctor tells him of his poor prognosis.

Mr Robinson complains of itching which is making him uncomfortable.

2 What causes this pruritus and what measures can the nurse take to relieve his discomfort?

During a conversation with the nurse Mr Robinson asks her to be a witness to his last will and testament and expresses a wish to donate his body to medical science.

3 What should be the nurse's response to Mr Robinson's request?

One evening following supper Mr Robinson has a massive haematemesis. The doctor passes a Sengstaken tube and prepares to administer two units of whole blood.

4 How would you explain the purpose of the tube to a junior nurse?

5   Identify, giving reasons, the specific nursing actions that would be implemented following passage of the tube.

Two days after Mr Robinson's haemorrhage you notice that he appears lethargic, tired and disorientated. His handwriting is becoming almost illegible and he has difficulty in solving simple addition and subtraction problems.

---

6   Explain the significance of these observations.
7   Giving reasons, explain how Mr Robinson's diet will be altered following the onset of these symptoms.
8   With reference to normal and altered physiology what would you tell a junior nurse about:
(a) cirrhosis of the liver?
(b) the cause of Mr Robinson's ascites and oesophageal varices?

5.3 Answers

1 Several views exist on how individuals react to the knowledge of impending death, however far away it may be. Probably the best known view is that of Dr Elizabeth Kubler-Ross.

- **Stage I—denial and isolation** Mr Robinson will probably initially deny that he is going to die. This stage is normal and gives the individual time to adopt coping strategies. He may continue to refuse to contact his sister because he denies the inevitable. He may isolate himself, i.e. draw into himself, and may feel very lonely, especially as he has no close relatives.
- **Stage II—anger** At some stage he is likely to acknowledge the threat of death as real. A natural reaction following this seems to be anger, rage, resentment and envy—'Why me?' Any members of the caring team may be the target of this anger. He may become aggressive or complaining and be difficult to care for.
- **Stage III—bargaining** Mr Robinson is beginning to accept his fate but is playing for time.
- **Stage IV—depression** His feelings of anger, resentment and envy are replaced by a sense of loss and he is likely to become depressed.
- **Stage V—acceptance** The final stage—the reality is faced and he is prepared to die. He may well wish to inform his sister of his illness.

2 Pruritus is caused by an accumulation of bile salts in the tissues. The bile salts accumulate because they are unable to be excreted by the damaged liver.

Measures for the relief of pruritus include:
- the application of something cold to cause vasoconstriction.
- soaking in the bath where possible. Add bath oils to the water.
- the use of cool, non-restrictive bed clothing.
- encouraging Mr Robinson to keep his nails short to avoid skin excoriation from scratching.
- the application of creams/medications, e.g. Calamine lotion.
- keeping room cool and humid.
- administering Questran, which increases the faecal excretion of bile salts.

3 It is inadvisable for a nurse to witness a will because of the

many complexities in doing so. The nurse should explain this and then advise Mr Robinson to contact a solicitor. The medical social worker may be able to help in this matter if necessary. If Mr Robinson does not want to wait this long the hospital administrator should be contacted. Explain to Mr Robinson that it may be quite possible for him to donate his body to medical science but that he needs to follow the correct procedure. Inform the hospital administrator who will indicate where Mr Robinson should send for a form.

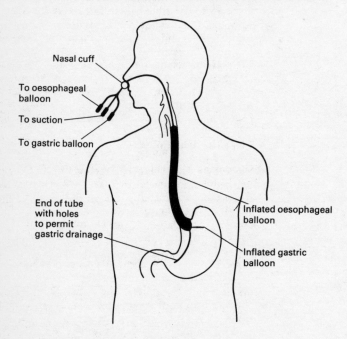

Fig. 10 The Sengstaken tube in situ.

4   • Find out how much the student knows.
    • Draw her the above diagram.
    • Explain that the inflated balloon exerts direct pressure on the bleeding varices in the lower oesophagus and upper stomach.

5

Nursing action	Rationale
Ensure that each lumen of the tube is correctly labelled.	This prevents possible error in inflation or deflation of the tube.
Observe Mr Robinson closely for any signs of respiratory distress.	As the oesophagus is obstructed by the tube Mr Robinson will not be able to swallow his saliva.
Provide Mr Robinson with a bowl for expectoration and tissues. Provide for suctioning his upper airway.	Provision must therefore be made to remove secretions.
Carry out intermittent gastic aspiration as directed by the doctor.	This removes blood from the stomach. If it is not removed the blood begins to break down and ammonia accumulates to toxic levels.
Deflate the balloons as ordered by the doctor.	This may be requested to reduce the possibility of tissue damage.
Keep Mr Robinson at rest.	This avoids displacement of the balloons.
Monitor the pulse and blood pressure. Check the pressures in the balloons as ordered.	This enables evaluation of the condition and bleeding, and ensures the maintenance of correct pressures.

6 The observations are indicative of the onset of hepatic encephalopathy. This is caused by failure of the liver to metabolize nitrogenous substances, e.g. ammonia. If treatment is not introduced promptly, Mr Robinson may lapse into a coma.

7 Restriction or elimination of dietary protein is essential to prevent the increase in the amount of accumulated ammonia (the breakdown product of protein). Before this, Mr Robinson's diet would have been high in protein. Following the onset of the symptoms he should also have a low sodium/high calorie diet to prevent ascites and provide glucose to prevent hypoglycaemia.

8 Normal physiology
Find out what the student already knows. Using previous

knowledge outline the structure and functions of the liver. Draw a diagram to show the blood supply to the liver (see Fig. 11).

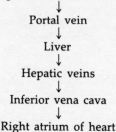

Fig. 11   The portal circulation.

Altered physiology

(a) Cirrhosis is a chronic liver disease in which diffuse destruction of hepatic cells has occurred followed by an increase in fibrous tissue formation. This fibrous tissue distorts the normal structure of the liver, leading to severe physiological abnormalities.

There are four major types of cirrhosis. The one associated with chronic abuse of alcohol is called Laennec's cirrhosis. Alcohol has a direct toxic effect on the liver cells which induces fatty infiltration of the liver. This eventually leads to cellular necrosis and fibrosis.

(b) The main factor contributing to both ascites and oesophageal varices is portal hypertension.

The pressure in the portal vein is increased by an obstruction of blood flow through the liver by the distorted liver cells. When the pressure is increased and the passage of blood through the liver is blocked, collateral channels develop to compensate. As these become distended with blood, the vessels enlarge and varices develop.

Increased pressure within the portal system increases the hydrostatic pressure within the veins. This increases the amount of fluid moved into the peritoneal cavity, leading to ascites. Another factor that contributes to the formation of ascites is decreased plasma albumin, which leads to reduced osmotic pressure.

Further Reading

General nursing

Brunner, L. & Suddarth, D. (1982) *The Lippincott Manual of Medical–Surgical Nursing*, Vol. 1–3. London: Harper & Row.

Clark, J.E., Sage, C.A. & Attree, M.J. (1985) *Revise Essential Nursing Care*, Letts Study Aids. London: Charles Letts & Co.

Faulkner, A. (1985) *Nursing—A Creative Approach*. London: Baillière Tindall.

Hunt, P. & Sendell, B. (1984) *Nursing the Adult with a Specific Physiological Disturbance*. London: The Macmillan Press.

Long, B.C. & Phipps, W.J. (1985) *Essentials of Medical–Surgical Nursing*. St Louis: C.V. Mosby.

Parkin, D. (1985) *Revise Nursing RGN*, Letts Study Aids. London: Charles Letts & Co.

Roper, N., Logan, W. & Tierney, A. (1985) *The Elements of Nursing*. Edinburgh: Churchill Livingstone.

The Royal Marsden Hospital (1984) In Pritchard, A. & Walker, V.A. (eds.) *Manual of Clinical Nursing Policies and Procedures*. London: Harper & Row.

Specific to topics included in this book

Dobree, J.H. & Boulter, E. (1982) *Blindness and Visual Handicap*. Oxford: Oxford University Press.

Garrett, G. (1983) *Health Needs of the Elderly*. London: The Macmillan Press.

Lerner, J. & Khan, Z. (1982) *Manual of Urological Nursing*. St Louis: C.V. Mosby.

Reynolds, M. (1984) *Gynaecological Nursing*. Oxford: Blackwell Scientific Publications.

Robbins, J. (1983) *Caring for the Dying Patient and Family*. London: Harper and Row.

Sutcliffe, T.H. (1984) *Deafness—Let's Face it*. London: Royal National Institute for the Deaf.